S0-CFE-865

There is no such thing as a perfect parent; we all learn to become the best parent we can be.

S.M. Gross

SIMPLEST PRESENTS

THE SIMPLEST PREGNANCY BOOK IN THE WORLD

Copyright © 2023 Simplest Company LLC.

All rights reserved.

All the text and artwork in this book are copyright © 2023 Simplest Company LLC. This book or any portion there of may not be reproduced, stored in a retrieval system, or transmitted, in any form or by any means, electronic, mechanical, photocopying, recording or distributing any part of it in any form without prior written permission from the publisher.

Printed in China

First printing May 2023

Paperback ISBN: 978-1-736894-79-8

Library of Congress Control Number: 2023909101

To order additional copies of the this book or for volume purchases and resale Send inquiries to: info@simplestbaby.com

Published by Simplest Company

Los Angeles, CA

simplestbaby.com

Illustrations by Stephen Gross

Copyright © 2023 Simplest Company LLC.

Simplest, Simplest Baby and Simplest Pregnancy are trademarks of Simplest Company LLC.

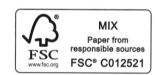

NOTE: The content of this book is for informational purposes only. The author, publisher and each individual who has made a contribution to the development and production of this book and its contents do not intend this book to be used as medical or other professional advice, and the book is not intended as a substitute for consultation with a licensed practitioner. This book is not intended to replace advice given to you by your and/or your child's physician, and any decisions concerning care are between you and your and/or your child's doctor. Please consult with your or your child's physician or healthcare specialist regarding the suggestions made in this book The publisher, the author and each individual who has made a contribution to the development and production of this book and its contents make no representations or warranties of any kind with respect to this book or its contents, and disclaim all such representations and warranties, express or implied. The examples provided in this book may not apply to the average reader, and are not intended to represent or guarantee that you will achieve the same or similar results. The publisher, the author each individual who has made a contribution to the development and production of this book and its contents assume no responsibility for errors, inaccuracies, omissions, or any other inconsistencies herein, and your use of this book implies your acceptance of this disclaimer.

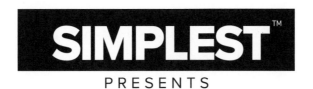

PRESENTS

THE
SIMPLEST™
PREGNANCY
BOOK IN THE WORLD

You Got This!
The Illustrated, Grab-and-Do Guide
for a Healthy, Happy Pregnancy
and Childbirth

S.M. Gross

Jeremy F. Shapiro, MD, MPH, FAAP

Natalia C. Llarena, MD, FACOG

Gabriella Terhes Karlsson, Newborn Care Specialist/Doula
& Sleep Trainer

and the Simplest Baby Community

KUDOS

How can a guy write a book on pregnancy?

It's a good question—one I asked myself when it was first proposed to me.

The short answer is: in some ways I didn't—moms, surrogates, doulas, female doctors, experts, and you did. My role was simply to curate, distill, design, and illustrate an incredible wealth of knowledge and know-how and create what is a super simple and practical resource that provides the fundamentals to make your journey far easier and joyful.

Kudos to the hundreds of moms and dads who shared their pregnancy stories— openly sharing their joys, challenges, and sorrows. Confiding with the many expecting parents who will read this book, your practical advice and clever workarounds will help sooooo many people. We very much appreciate you and your contribution.

Kudos to the very special surrogate moms whose participation in this book provided an invaluable perspective that other moms-to-be will find tremendously helpful. Also, I want to personally say how grateful I am for the wonder you brought to my life with our amazing children.

Kudos to the incredible team of individuals who shared so generously their knowledge, experiences, and time. We are so fortunate to have worked with such a broad range of talented individuals who have a passion for helping expectant moms and dads and their babies. You are truly inspiring.

To those who supported the efforts and encouraged the team along the way, thank you!

OUR STORY

What was born out of necessity—to find the simple, practical solutions and information for parenting—has proven to resonate with today's moms and dads. Our first book, *The Simplest Baby Book In The World,* has been a success since day one and has reinvented the way parenting information is created and shared for today's generation.

It quickly became clear that the same desire for simplicity—focusing on proven basics and practical fundamentals—that parents yearned for in the first year of raising a baby is even more needed in the complicated and stressful nine months of pregnancy. Becoming pregnant for the first time is a source of great excitement and joy, but it can also be a time filled with anxiety and stress due to the complex nature of pregnancy and the multitude of questions that arise throughout one's journey.

We found the information out there—books, websites, blogs, videos, and so on—all too dense, overwhelming, and not simple enough to meet today's needs. There is certainly no lack of information—in fact, there is too much! On a daily basis we are all inundated by a seemingly endless number of voices that make it hard to parse through and identify the best solutions.

So, we did a lot of research; we held countless conversations with the community of those who know best—doctors, OB-GYNs, nurses, surrogates, nannies, doulas, midwives, educators, other moms and dads, among others—and distilled that knowledge down to its essentials. And that is how the idea for the *Simplest Pregnancy* book was born: the desire to share this collective knowledge and advice in a way that provides parents-to-be with practical information and solutions they can find quickly and easily.

DON'T PANIC.
YOU GOT THIS

WHY YOU NEED THIS BOOK

For this book, I assume you:

- Are pregnant or are planning to be.

- Are interested in learning to take good care of yourself.

- Want to have a healthy pregnancy and baby.

- Don't have time to go through 600-plus-page books.

- Are tired of getting random information from friends, family, and the internet.

- Want to buy what you *really* need and not overspend.

- Want recommendations on the best products.

- Want to take control of your life.

- Want your partner to understand pregnancy.

- Want to spend more time enjoying your pregnancy journey.

SIMPLEST PREGNANCY
HOW IT WORKS

1. START WITH THE BIG PICTURE AND GET ORGANIZED

An overview of getting pregnant and some of the first things you're going to want to do for a smooth pregnancy.

2. TRACK TRIMESTER BY TRIMESTER DEVELOPMENTS

A walk through each trimester and the key things that happen in each of them, so you are well prepared.

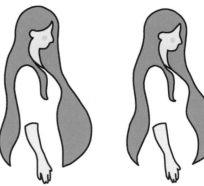

1 Trimester　　**2 Trimester**　　**3 Trimester**

AND GET FREE SIMPLEST™

QR Codes activate FREE content

Scan the QR codes throughout the book for quick access to **FREE** additional must-have, grab-and-do resources, organizing tools, and planners that complement the book and make the journey just a little easier.

TIPS & SHORTCUTS

Sprinkled throughout the book you will find these helpful tips.

 QUICK TIP Small, practical, expert recommendations that help make life just a little easier.

 Mommy Hack Mom's simple solutions and clever workarounds for everyday pregnancy issues.

3. PREPARE FOR LABOR, DELIVERY, AND RECOVERY

What can happen during labor, delivery, and your postpartum recovery.

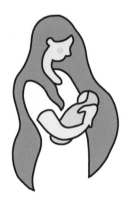

PLUS

LEARN THE ESSENTIALS YOU NEED TO KNOW

Topics include:

 Nutrition

 Safety

 Health

 Mental Health

ESSENTIAL TOOLS!

 Pregnancy Planner and Tracker

 Must-Haves Checklists by Trimester

 Birth Plan Builder

 Hospital Bag Essentials

 Baby Shower Planner

and so much more!

CONTENTS

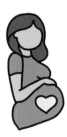

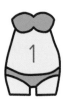

THIRD TRIMESTER
What happens in weeks 28 to 40 to your body and to baby. Preparing your birth plan, hospital bag, pain-management plan, childbirth classes, breast pumps, false labor, bump support, water breaking, symptoms, and more.

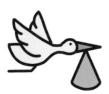

DELIVERY
The stages of labor, contractions, effacement, labor positions, types of delivery, birthing positions, premature births, as well as overdue and induced births.

ARRIVAL
Time to celebrate and learn about skin-to-skin contact, baby's first feedings, and the types of screenings done upon baby's delivery.

RECOVERY
The essentials of the postpartum period from lochia, and various other symptoms, to getting back in shape, sex, and all the possible aspects.

SAFETY
A primer on the various risks to you and your baby, as well as tips on how to prepare the nursery.

HEALTH CONCERNS
Key health concerns and complications—what they are and how to prevent and treatment them.

MENTAL HEALTH
Having a baby brings up many emotions, from depression and anger to guilt for mom and dad; learn how to handle them.

Something
wonderful is
about
to happen.

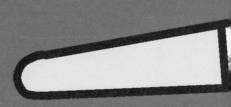

PREGNANCY OVERVIEW

Understanding the big picture and how it all happens.

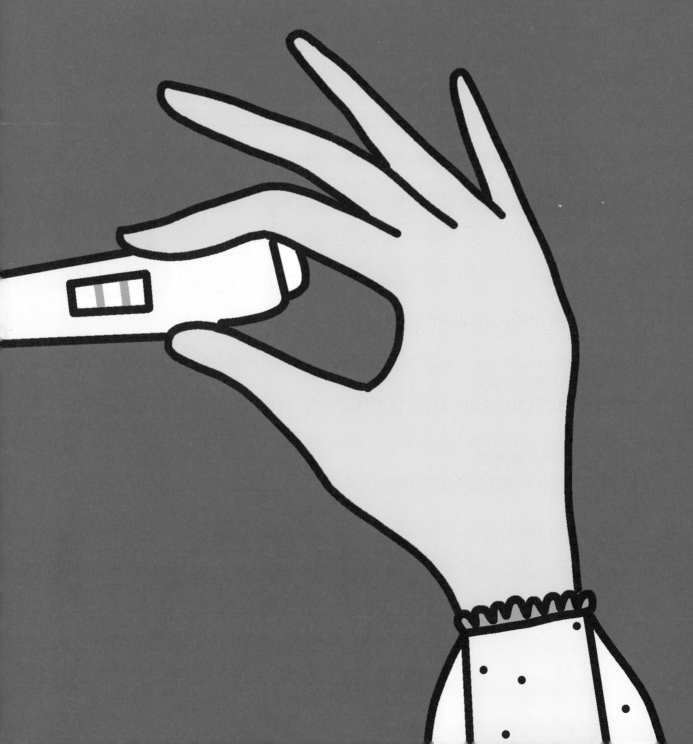

PREGNANCY
OVERVIEW

WHAT IS IT?

PREGNANCY: The condition or period of time in which a fetus grows and develops inside a woman's womb or uterus.

HOW LONG DOES IT LAST?

A normal, full-term pregnancy lasts approximately 40 weeks from the first day of the last menstrual period (LMP). Because pregnancies are dated by the LMP, an extra two weeks are included at the beginning of pregnancy before conception actually occurs. That is why pregnancy lasts 40 weeks (approx. 10 months) rather than nine months.

A NORMAL PREGNANCY LASTS **40**WEEKS OR 10 MONTHS

1st TRIMESTER
0–13 WEEKS: MONTHS 1–3

2nd TRIMESTER
14–27 WEEKS: MONTHS 4–7

3rd TRIMESTER
28–40 WEEKS: MONTHS 7–10

HOW DOES IT HAPPEN?

To become pregnant, a sperm needs to fertilize an egg; this is called fertilization. Pregnancy officially begins when the fertilized egg implants in the wall of the uterus; implantation occurs five to seven days after fertilization.

METHODS OF CONCEPTION

There are two methods of conception:

1. SEXUAL INTERCOURSE

The physical act of intercourse (the insertion of a penis into a vagina), resulting in the ejaculation of semen into the vagina.

2. ASSISTED REPRODUCTION

Conception achieved through any means other than intercourse. There are two main categories of assisted reproduction: artificial insemination and in vitro fertilization.

A. ARTIFICIAL INSEMINATION

A fertility method used to deliver sperm directly to the cervix or uterus.

1. Intrauterine Insemination (IUI)

Sperm is injected directly into the uterus by a health-care provider.

2. Intra-cervical Insemination (ICI)

Sperm is injected into the cervix (the area just outside the uterus); it can be done at home by you or in office by a health-care provider.

B. IN VITRO FERTILIZATION (IVF)

Eggs are removed from the woman and are fertilized outside her body, and an embryo is placed back in her uterus.

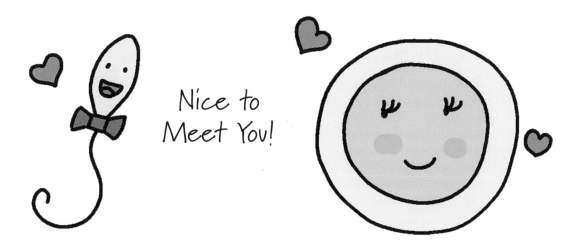

Nice to Meet You!

STAGES OF PREGNANCY

THE TIMELINE FOR PREGNANCY

Pregnancy is broken into three trimesters. An additional fourth trimester begins after birth.

1st TRIMESTER (WEEKS 0–13)

The first trimester is the phase of pregnancy that begins at conception and lasts for 13 weeks or three months. The first trimester is counted from the first day of your last period. This is a bit odd, but it's done this way because most women won't know the exact date of conception.

GERMINAL STAGE • FIRST 14 DAYS

The first 14-day or two-week period during which the fertilized egg travels to the uterus, dividing and multiplying until it implants in the lining of the uterus.

EMBRYONIC STAGE • WEEKS 3–10

This stage begins at the start of the third week after conception. Many changes occur during this time. The cells continue to divide, and the various major organs begin to take shape.

FETAL STAGE • WEEK 11–BIRTH

At this stage the baby is called a fetus. During this stage, amazing development and growth occur.

2nd TRIMESTER (WEEKS 14–27)

During this period, many of the unpleasant effects of the first trimester have somewhat subsided.

STAGES OF PREGNANCY

1st TRIMESTER	2nd TRIMESTER	3rd TRIMESTER

GERMINAL STAGE	← EMBRYONIC STAGE →	← FETAL STAGE →

3rd TRIMESTER (WEEKS 28–UNTIL BIRTH)

This is the final stage before birth. Your fetus will continue to grow in size and weight, and the baby will start to move into position for delivery.

4th TRIMESTER (POSTPARTUM)

Refers to the 12 weeks or three-month period directly following delivery. It is the time when mom recovers and the baby adjusts to no longer being in the womb.

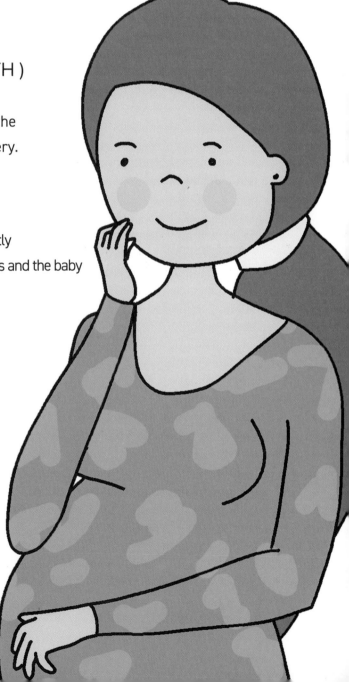

PREGNANCY TIMELINE

WHAT TO DO AND WHEN

Every pregnancy is different, but what follows is a general timeline of some of the key dates, activities, and milestones during a healthy, uncomplicated pregnancy.

WEEKS 1 2 3 4 5 6 7 8 9 10 11 12 13 14 15 16 17 18

Baby

Technically
PREGNANT

Hearing
BABY'S HEARTBEAT

TOES
developing

TEETH BUDS
start forming

FLUTTERS
Feel baby
movement

Medical

3 months
ahead of pregnancy
PRENATAL VITAMINS

Schedule
PRENATAL APPT.

MORNING SICKNESS
Begins

First
PRENATAL VISIT

First
ULTRASOUND

BRAXTON HICKS

Second
PRENATAL VISIT

Paperwork
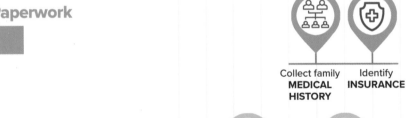

Collect family
MEDICAL HISTORY

Identify
INSURANCE

Other Stuff

Identify
CHILDCARE

Plan
MATERNITY LEAVE

First
BUMP PHOTO

Sharing
I'M PREGNANT

Set up
BABY REGISTRY

WEEKS 1 2 3 4 5 6 7 8 9 10 11 12 13 14 15 16 17 18

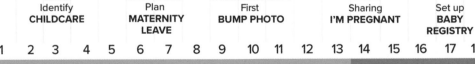

1st TRIMESTER   **2nd T**

← 40 WE

GET YOUR <u>FREE</u> INDISPENSABLE PREGNANCY PLANNER AND TRACKER:

Scan this QR code for easy access to get our comprehensive pregnancy tracker, baby weekly developmental milestones, and weekly to dos, so you forget nothing.

20 21 22 23 24 25 26 27 28 29 30 31 32 33 34 35 36 37 38 39 40

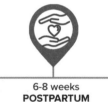

ning
S SEX

Baby response to
YOUR VOICE

EYES
are Light
Sensitive

BABY SKIN
is becoming
opaque

LUNGS
fully developed

cond
SOUND

First
3D
ULTRASOUND

Considered
FULL TERM

6-8 weeks
POSTPARTUM
RECOVERY

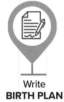

Write
BIRTH PLAN

Collect documents for
HOSPITAL

Preregister at
HOSPITAL

cond
PHOTO

Planning
NURSERY

Brainstorm
BABY NAMES

CHILDBIRTH
CLASS

Third
BUMP
PHOTO

Pack
HOSPITAL
BAG

BABY
SHOWER

Complete
NURSERY

20 21 22 23 24 25 26 27 28 29 30 31 32 33 34 35 36 37 38 39 40

MESTER **3rd TRIMESTER**

- 280 DAYS ⟶

CONCEPTION
YOU'RE ON YOUR WAY

The who, what, and how of conception.

WHAT IS IT?

CONCEPTION: Also known as fertilization, it is the merging of a sperm and egg. It is the first step toward pregnancy.

HOW LONG DOES IT TAKE?

In most cases, conception occurs in a woman's fallopian tube within hours or days after sexual intercourse. This is not the case with IVF.

QUICK TIP

A woman can still get pregnant five days after having sex, because the sperm can live up to five days in a woman's body.

HOW LONG DO EGGS & SPERM LIVE?

AN EGG'S LIFESPAN = **12 to 24 Hours** AFTER OVULATION

A SPERM'S LIFESPAN = **5 Days**

FROM EGG TO FETUS

SPERM

The male reproductive cell or gamete.

EGG

The egg, or ovum, is the female reproductive cell or gamete. It is one of the largest cells in the human body.

FERTILIZATION

The successful joining of an egg and sperm to form the primary nucleus of the embryo. This can happen within hours or days after sex.

ZYGOTE

The single cell formed by the successful merging of an egg and sperm.

BLASTOCYST

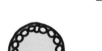

This phase of development happens between five and nine days after fertilization. It is now a multi-cell cluster from which the inner cell mass becomes the embryo and the outer cell layer becomes the placenta.

EMBRYO

An early stage in the development of a human egg cell. By the end of the eight-week embryonic period, 90 percent of the adult structure has formed.

FETUS

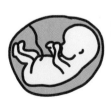

Eleven weeks after fertilization, the embryo, having formed the basic structure of a human, is considered a fetus.

AN EGG'S JOURNEY
INSEMINATION TO IMPLANTATION

The time frame from ovulation to implantation takes about six to ten days.

 OVARIES
The eggs are produced and stored in the ovaries until they are ready to be released.

 INSEMINATION
You have done the deed either via sex or artificial insemination.

SPERM
The sperm now travels from the vagina to the cervix. The cervical mucus functions like a nightclub doorman, only letting in the best of the group.

 OVULATION
An egg is released from the ovaries and travels down the fallopian tube, where it will stay for 12 to 24 hours.

 FERTILIZATION
The sperm has continued on its journey, now going up the fallopian tube, where it meets and merges with the egg.

 ZYGOTE
Once the egg and sperm merge, it becomes a zygote.

 BLASTOCYST
The zygote begins traveling down the fallopian tube, all the while dividing. When it reaches the uterus, it becomes a blastocyst.

 IMPLANTATION
The blastocyst now implants itself into the lining of the uterus, where it will stay until delivery begins.

HOW IT HAPPENS

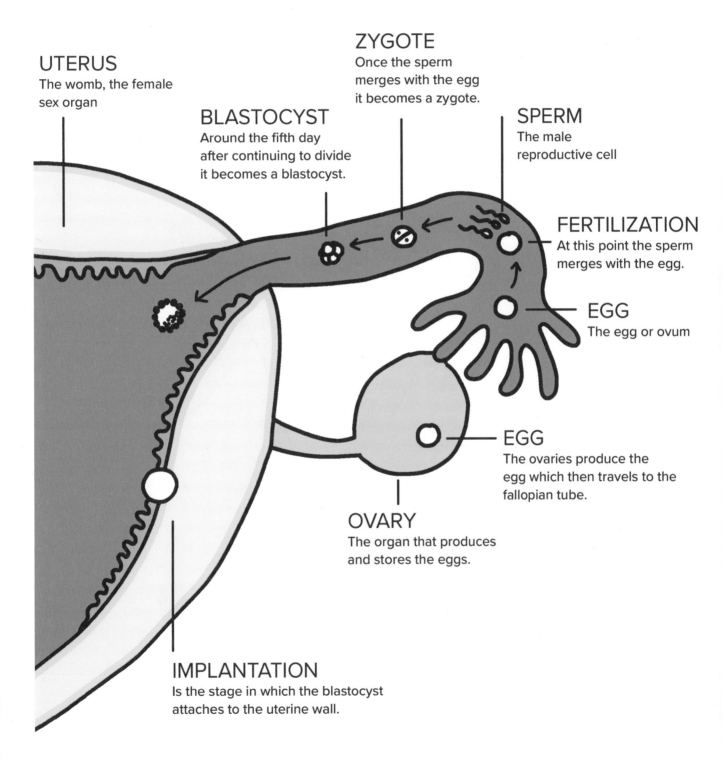

UTERUS
The womb, the female sex organ

BLASTOCYST
Around the fifth day after continuing to divide it becomes a blastocyst.

ZYGOTE
Once the sperm merges with the egg it becomes a zygote.

SPERM
The male reproductive cell

FERTILIZATION
At this point the sperm merges with the egg.

EGG
The egg or ovum

EGG
The ovaries produce the egg which then travels to the fallopian tube.

OVARY
The organ that produces and stores the eggs.

IMPLANTATION
Is the stage in which the blastocyst attaches to the uterine wall.

EMBRYO DEVELOPMENT
BECOMING A BABY

What happens once the egg is implanted in the lining of the uterus?

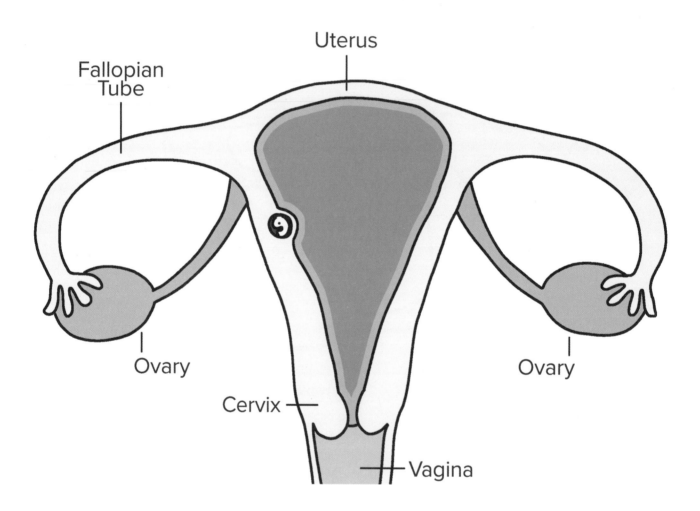

WHAT NOW?

After implantation of the blastocyst in the lining of the uterus, it will continue to develop, forming into a fetus, placenta, and amniotic sac.

EMBRYONIC & FETAL DEVELOPMENT

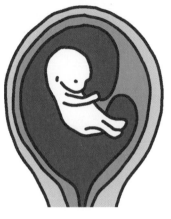

9 WEEKS

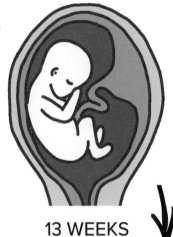

13 WEEKS

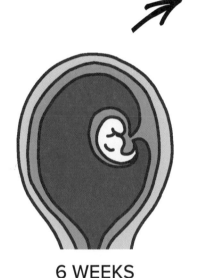

6 WEEKS

DEVELOPMENT OF THE EMBRYO & FETUS

In the embryonic stage of development, the baby's internal organs and its external body structures are formed. During the fetal period, the organs continue to develop and grow larger in size until delivery.

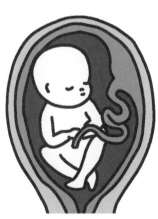

20 WEEKS

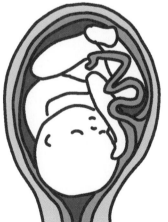

38–40 WEEKS

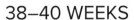

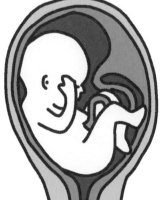

27 WEEKS

PLACENTA
WE HAVE A REAL CONNECTION

Everything you need to know about the placenta.

WHAT IS IT?

PLACENTA: The placenta is a temporary fetal organ that develops after the egg implants itself at the top or side of the lining of the uterus. The placenta, via an umbilical cord, connects the mother to baby.

WHAT DOES IT DO?

The placenta plays a critical role in the development of baby; it literally reprograms mom's body to help in the development of the baby. It ensures that the mother's blood does not mix with the baby's blood by filtering it and allowing only the transfer of:

- Oxygen, and removal of carbon dioxide;

- Nutrients and water;

- Hormones for mother and baby;

- Antibodies, which offer some immunity to baby when it is born;

- Drugs, if needed, for baby's development.

WHAT HAPPENS TO IT?

The placenta is expelled from the uterus after the baby is delivered.

TIPS FOR A HEALTHY PLACENTA

- Remain active, go on walks, practice meditation and breathing exercises.

- Manage your blood pressure.

- Avoid stress.

- Keep or get up to date on vaccinations recommended for pregnancy.

- Sleep on your side.

- Avoid high-altitude travel that might reduce your oxygen supply.

A HEALTHY PLACENTA

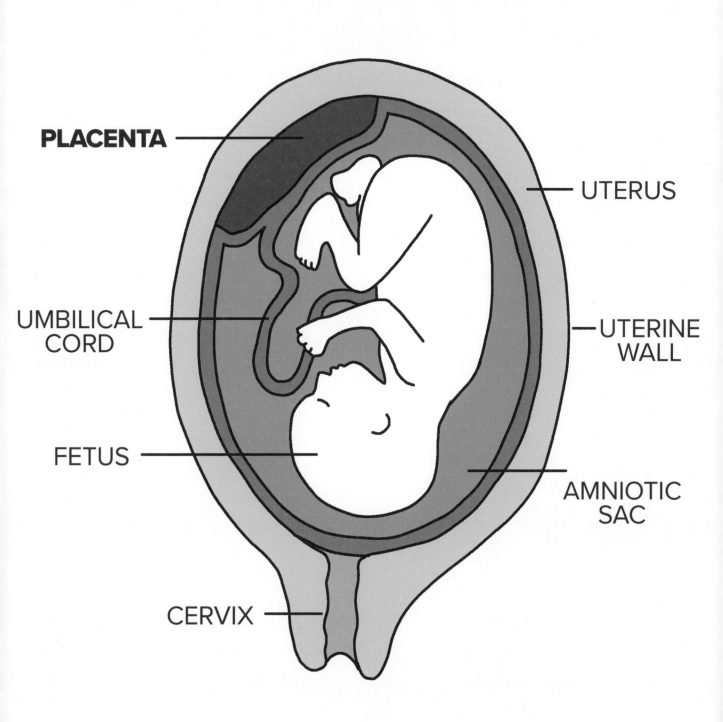

PLACENTA

UTERUS

UMBILICAL CORD

UTERINE WALL

FETUS

AMNIOTIC SAC

CERVIX

TYPES OF PREGNANCIES

NOT ALL PREGNANCIES ARE THE SAME

You'll hear different terms used to describe the various types of pregnancies. Here is a breakdown of what they all mean.

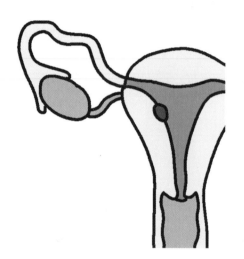

NORMAL PREGNANCY
(Intrauterine Pregnancy)

Occurs when the egg implants in the upper side of the lining of the uterus and the placenta attaches normally.

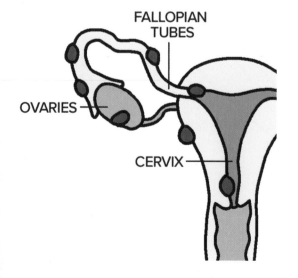

FALLOPIAN TUBES

OVARIES

CERVIX

ECTOPIC PREGNANCY

Occurs when the fertilized egg implants outside the cavity of the uterus. These pregnancies are not viable and require you to see your doctor for evaluation and treatment. It could implant in:

- The ovaries
- The lower section of the uterus (cervix)
- The fallopian tubes (**Tubal Pregnancy**)
- The abdominal cavity (**Intra-Abdominal Pregnancy**): where the fetus grows into the abdominal cavity.

NOTE: Always speak to your health-care provider about what to expect with any health or pregnancy issues to understand the risks and benefits so that you and your baby are kept safe.

SINGLETON PREGNANCY

Occurs when a single egg meets a single sperm and produces one fetus.

MULTIPLE PREGNANCY

Occurs when you are carrying more than one baby at a time.

TWINS: Carrying two babies.

IDENTICAL TWINS: Twins that occur when a single egg is fertilized by one sperm and divides into two zygotes.

FRATERNAL TWINS: Occur when two eggs are fertilized at the same time by two separate sperm.

TRIPLETS: Carrying three babies.

QUADRUPLETS: Carrying four babies.

QUINTUPLETS: Carrying five babies.

HIGH-RISK PREGNANCY

Pregnancies that have an increased risk of complications; may occur, for example, if birth parent:

- Is over the age of 35.
- Is a teenager.
- Has diabetes.
- Overweight or obese.
- Has had multiple pregnancy.
- Fetus has birth defects.
- Has other health conditions that affect the pregnancy.
- Takes medication to control a medical condition.
- Has a history of pregnancies with complications or preterm birth.

CHEMICAL PREGNANCY

Occurs when an egg is fertilized and implanted but stops developing within the first five weeks, resulting in a very early miscarriage.

MOLAR PREGNANCY

When an egg and sperm fertilize incorrectly and form a noncancerous tumor. Molar pregnancies require early treatment. They can result in serious complications.

Complete Molar: An abnormal placenta forms, but without a baby/fetus.

Partial Molar: Normal or abnormal placenta tissue forms, and a nonviable fetus may also form.

HOW BIG IS MY BABY?

Curious about the size of baby? Well, to give you an idea, in this chart we compare your baby's size to common fruits, nuts, and vegetables throughout the weeks of your pregnancy.

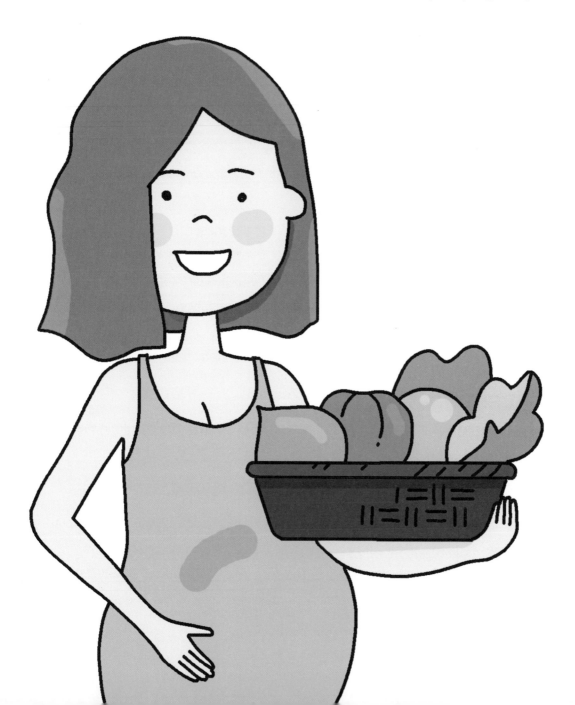

SIZE COMPARISON CHART

 WEEK 4
POPPY SEED

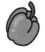 **WEEK 5**
APPLE SEED

 WEEK 6
LENTIL

 WEEK 7
BLUEBERRY

 WEEK 8
RASPBERRY

 WEEK 9
GRAPE

 WEEK 10
PEANUT

 WEEK 11
FIG

 WEEK 12
PLUM

 WEEK 13
LEMON

 WEEK 14
PEACH

 WEEK 15
APPLE

 WEEK 16
AVOCADO

 WEEK 17
PEAR

WEEK 18
BELL PEPPER

WEEK 19
BIG TOMATO

WEEK 20
ARTICHOKE

WEEK 21
CARROT

WEEK 22
MANGO

WEEK 23
GRAPEFRUIT

WEEK 24
CORN

WEEK 25
RUTABAGA

WEEK 26
LETTUCE

WEEK 27
CAULIFLOWER

WEEK 28
EGGPLANT

 WEEK 29
ACORN SQUASH

 WEEK 30
CABBAGE

 WEEK 31
COCONUT

 WEEK 32
PINEAPPLE

 WEEK 33
BUTTERNUT SQUASH

 WEEK 34
HONEYDEW MELON

 WEEK 35
SWISS CHARD

 WEEK 36
HEAD OF ROMAINE

 WEEK 37
LENGTH OF A LEEK

 WEEK 38
WINTER MELON

 WEEK 39
PUMPKIN

 WEEK 40
WATERMELON

SIGNS OF PREGNANCY

HOW DO I KNOW I'M PREGNANT?

Every person is different and experiences the symptoms of pregnancy differently.

QUICK TIP

If you have missed your period, the best way to know if you are pregnant is to take a pregnancy test.

WHEN DO THEY START?

Typically, you may begin experiencing symptoms one to two weeks after conception. However, many of the symptoms are similar to common occurrences, such as coming down with a cold and the beginning of your period. Some women have no symptoms at all.

WHAT CAUSES IT?

Most of the early signs of pregnancy are due to the release of the human chorionic gonadotropin hormone (hCG) and progesterone.

COMMON SIGNS OF PREGNANCY

MISSED PERIOD

The most common sign of pregnancy is a missed period. If a week or more has passed since your regular menstrual start date, you might be pregnant. However, you could be experiencing an irregular menstrual cycle.

CHANGES IN YOUR BREASTS

Hormonal changes cause your breasts to become swollen and sore. Your breasts might feel heavier, fuller, and tingly, while your nipples might enlarge and become darker.

NAUSEA

Feeling nauseated, with or without throwing up, may start for some people as early as two weeks after conception. Often called morning sickness, it can happen at any time of day.

INCREASED URINATION

You may find yourself making more trips to the bathroom. This occurs because your body has produced more blood, resulting in more fluids being filtered by your kidneys.

FATIGUE

Feeling run-down and tired is one of the most reported symptoms of pregnancy. Elevated levels of the hormone progesterone result in sleeplessness and increased fatigue.

LESS COMMON SIGNS OF PREGNANCY

LIGHT SPOTTING

Small amount of bleeding, usually the result of implantation.

CRAMPING

Cramping, similar to when your period is starting.

BLOATING

Feeling bloated, similar to when starting your menstrual period.

MOOD SWINGS

Feeling emotional or weepy is very common.

FEELING HOT

Caused by increased body temperature.

HEADACHES

Increased blood flow may cause you to experience headaches.

CONSTIPATION

Caused by the digestive system slowing down, resulting in constipation.

FOOD CRAVINGS & AVERSIONS

Greater sensitivity to certain tastes and smells; craving some foods and utterly hating others.

DIZZINESS

Feeling of light-headedness.

PREGNANCY TESTS

THE TYPES OF TESTS

WHAT IS IT?

A pregnancy test determines if you are pregnant by checking for the hormone human chorionic gonadotropin (hCG) in your urine or blood. Found only in pregnant women, hCG is made by the placenta once an egg implants.

QUICK TIP

It's important to understand that digital pregnancy tests are worse for the environment than non-digital tests. Both are one-time use devices, but with a digital test, one ends up throwing out both the electronics and a battery.

TYPES OF TESTS

AT-HOME TESTS

There are two types of home pregnancy tests: **NON-DIGITAL** and **DIGITAL.** Both are very accurate in detecting pregnancy when used correctly. However, the non-digital test is slightly more sensitive.

1. HOME TEST (Non-digital)

A home non-digital pregnancy test (HPT) is used on the first day you miss your period. It works by detecting (hCG) in your urine.

Accuracy: High, when used correctly

Results: 10 minutes

Purchased: Local drug stores, grocery stores, and some convenience stores

2. HOME TEST (Digital)

A home digital pregnancy test (HPT) is used on the first day you miss your period. It works by detecting (hCG) in your urine.

Accuracy: High, when used correctly

Results: 3 minutes

Purchased: Local drug stores, grocery stores, and some convenience stores

CLINICAL URINE TEST

This test is similar to the home test, but it is performed by medical personnel.

Accuracy: High

Results: Within a week

Purchased: At a clinic or your doctor's office

BLOOD TESTS

Performed at a clinic or in the doctor's office, there are two types:

1. Qualitative hCG blood test, which checks for the production of hCG in the body.

   Accuracy: High

   Results: A couple of days

2. Quantitative hCG blood test, which measures the level of hCG in the blood.

   Accuracy: Extremely high

   Results: More than a week

PREGNANCY TEST URINE OR BLOOD IS
99% accurate

FALSE POSITIVE

False positives are very rare but can occur. Here are some reasons for a false positive:

RECENT MISCARRIAGE

MENOPAUSE

CERTAIN MEDICATIONS
Such as hCG, used for fertility treatments.

RARE FORM OF CANCER
In rare cases, certain forms of cancer can produce hCG (ovarian and gastrointestinal).

USER ERROR
Interpreting the test outside the recommended time interval.

FALSE NEGATIVE

False negative can occur. Here are some reasons for a false negative:

TEST TAKEN TOO EARLY
It is best taken a few days or a week after a missed period.

URINE IS TOO DILUTED

NOT WAITING 5 MIN. FOR RESULTS

PREGNANCY TESTS

HOME TEST: TYPICALLY HOW IT WORKS

HOME TEST (Non-Digital) • HOW IT WORKS

You will need to collect a urine sample. It's best if you collect the sample in the morning, as the urine is the most concentrated at that time of day; but you can take the test at any time of day.

Remove the test from the packaging. Place the point of the stick into the urine, and leave it there for the manufacturer's recommended duration. Next, remove it, and let it stand according to the instructions on the packaging.

TWO COLLECTION METHODS

1. Hold the test strip in your urine stream while sitting on the toilet.
2. Collect your urine in a clean cup. Then, dip the test strip into it.

NEGATIVE   **POSITIVE**

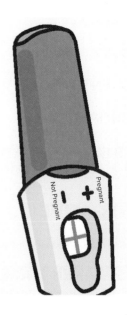

Most non-digital test strips use colored lines (color may vary depending on the brand) to show if you are pregnant.

HOME TEST (Digital) • HOW IT WORKS

You will need to collect a urine sample. It's best if you collect the sample in the morning, as the urine is the most concentrated at that time of day; but you can take the test at any time of day.

Remove the test from the packaging. Place the point of the stick into the urine, and leave it there for at least eight seconds. Next, remove it, and let it stand according to the instructions on the packaging.

TWO COLLECTION METHODS

1. Hold the test strip in your urine stream while sitting on the toilet.
2. Collect your urine in a clean cup. Then, dip the test strip into it.

If you are pregnant, most test strips show a colored line, which varies depending on the brand used.

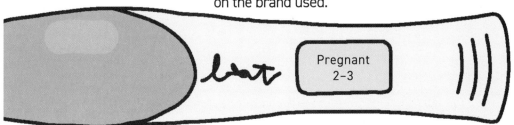

Depending on the brand, the negative or positive results are shown differently. For example, some simply read YES or NO, or give an estimate of how many weeks pregnant you are.

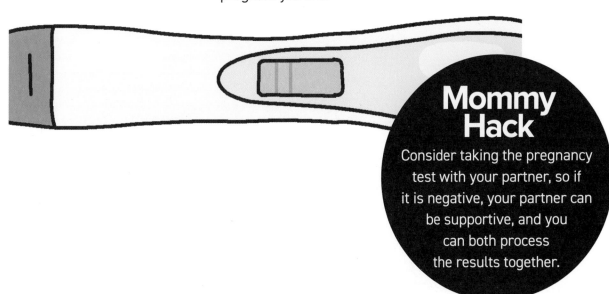

Mommy Hack

Consider taking the pregnancy test with your partner, so if it is negative, your partner can be supportive, and you can both process the results together.

Time to
get your
ducks
in a row.

GETTING ORGANIZED

Now that you are pregnant, what are the things that you need to do and know?

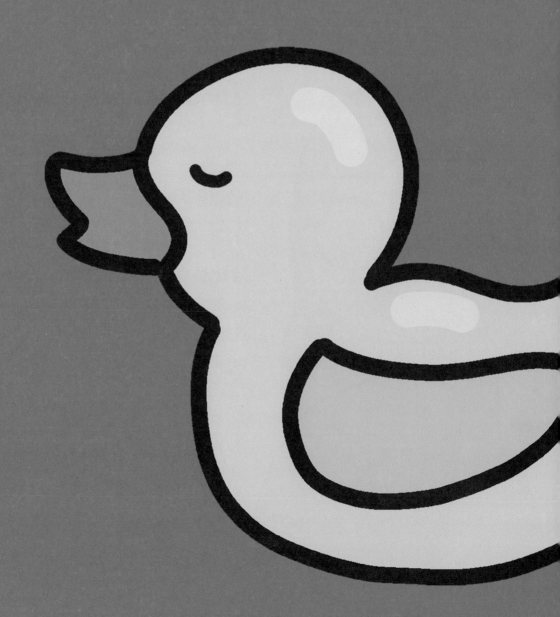

I'M PREGNANT!

WHAT NOW?

Learning you are pregnant can be a lot to take in, and figuring out what to do next can be overwhelming too. Not to worry, we've outlined some of the next steps for you. Right now, take a moment to enjoy this incredibly special moment.

WHAT TO DO WHEN YOU KNOW YOU'RE PREGNANT

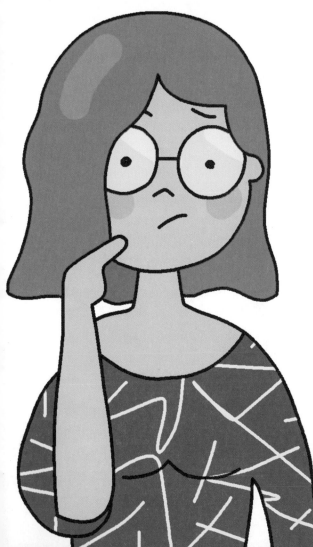

CHOOSE A HEALTH-CARE PROVIDER

Decide on a doctor or midwife who is a good match for you, and schedule an appointment.

TAKE PRENATAL VITAMINS

Take a vitamin with at least 400 mcg of folic acid daily.

STOP USING ALCOHOL OR DRUGS

Alcohol and drugs can cause serious damage to your baby's development.

STOP SMOKING

Smoking increases the chances of complications from exposure to harmful chemicals. Secondhand smoke can also be harmful to baby.

UNDERSTAND YOUR MEDICAL HISTORY

Pull together your family medical history, and your partner's, for your doctor.

SCHEDULE YOUR FIRST PRENATAL VISIT

Book your first prenatal visit on the books to confirm your pregnancy with an early ultrasound and blood work and to review your medical history.

AVOID THE PREGNANCY NO-NOs

Understand all the things that you should avoid during your pregnancy.

ACCESS YOUR DIET

Nutrition is critically important for you and baby, so eating the right foods is essential.

PREPARE FOR PREGNANCY SYMPTOMS

Everyone experiences pregnancy differently, but it is best to understand the potential changes that will be taking place in your body and the various symptoms that may occur.

MAKE A WORK PLAN

Decide how long you want to work. Check in with human resources to understand the company's maternity policy and benefits.

CHECK YOUR VACCINATION HISTORY

Make sure you are up to date on all your shots.

CENTER YOURSELF

Becoming pregnant can create a mix of emotions, from joy to sadness, happiness to depression. If you are struggling with these feelings, tell someone, so you can get help.

DECIDE WHEN AND WHOM TO TELL

Determine the best time and way to share the good news.

CHECK IN WITH YOUR DENTIST

Your body will be going through lots of changes; your teeth and gums are no exception.

CALCULATE YOUR DUE DATE

Understand what your due date and other key dates mean.

SURPRISE
TELLING YOUR PARTNER

You're so excited and bursting at the seams to share the great news with your partner, but you want to do it in a fun way. Here are some super cute and clever ideas.

CUTE ANNOUNCEMENT IDEAS

IT'S IN THE BAG

Mix baby diapers, baby food, or other baby items in with your regular groceries, and ask your partner to help you unpack them. "Surprise!"

LET YOUR PARTNER DISCOVER

Leave one or several (depending on how observant your partner is) pregnancy tests out on the bathroom counter for your partner to discover.

GOT MAIL

Send a birth announcement to your partner.

SPECIAL DELIVERY

Order your favorite baby book or a onesie that has a message on it, and send it to your partner.

BEEP BEEP BEEP

Place a bun in the oven and set the oven timer so that your partner is in the kitchen when it goes off. Ask your partner to take it out of the oven. Imagine your partner's surprise on seeing "a bun in the oven."

T-SHIRT

Give your partner a T-shirt with a special message, Dad- or Mom-To-Be, Best Dad Ever, etc.

LEAVE CLUES

Sprinkle around your home various baby things—a baby book, parenting magazines, a pacifier, or baby name books—for your partner to discover.

SERVE IT UP

Go out to dinner with your partner to a restaurant where you have prearranged for a dessert served on a plate with the message, "We are pregnant."

BABY SHOES

Hang a pair of baby shoes over your partner's rearview mirror.

SURPRISE DESSERT

Bake or give your partner a cake or cupcake with a special message on it.

EGG IT UP

Write a message on an egg. As you are cooking, ask your partner to get you a couple eggs from the refrigerator.

SPELL IT OUT

Leave a pregnancy message on the bathroom mirror for your partner to discover.

BELLY UP

Write a message on your belly that your partner will discover or that you reveal.

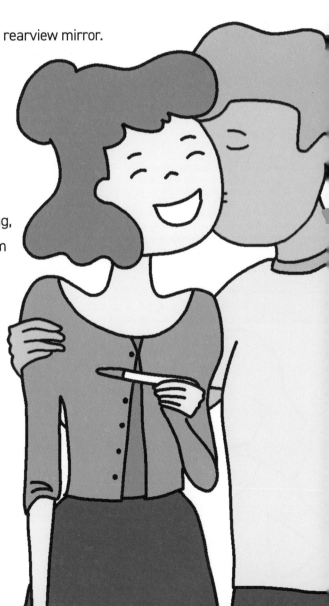

SHARING THE GOOD NEWS

HOW & WHEN

You're pregnant! When is the right time to share the happy news? Honestly, there is no specific right time; it's whenever you want to. Announcing your pregnancy is a personal decision—one that only you and your partner can make.

TELLING YOUR PARTNER

The first person you will more than likely tell is your partner.

You should get your partner's perspective on when and how to share the news and develop a plan based on input from both of you. If the pregnancy was unplanned, you and your partner might need to deal with your own emotions before telling anyone else.

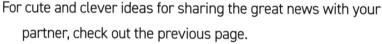

For cute and clever ideas for sharing the great news with your partner, check out the previous page.

QUICK TIP

If you have a friend who has been struggling with getting pregnant, you may want to tell them privately.

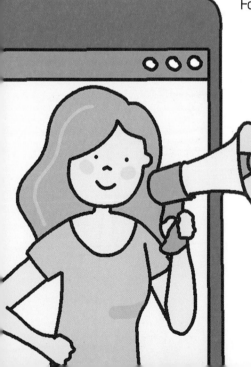

TYPICAL TIME PEOPLE SHARE THE NEWS

AFTER WEEK **12** • TRIMESTER **2ND**

Parents-to-be feel the most comfortable sharing the news at the beginning of the second trimester, because this period is widely considered the "safe zone," when the risk of miscarriage has diminished.

TELLING FAMILY & FRIENDS

Family

Consider telling your family first. Your pregnancy will be major news to them, especially the grandparents-to-be. They more than likely will want to celebrate with you.

Friends

Your closest friends will be among the first that you share the great news with. After telling your inner circle, social media might be your go-to place for making things more public.

TELLING YOUR EMPLOYER & COWORKERS

Coworkers and your boss are not typically at the top of the list, but sharing the news at work depends on several things. For example,

- If your job requires heavy lifting, exposure to chemicals, or other hazards.
- If you are going to be taking parental leave or time off from work.

In cases like these, you may tell your direct supervisor and decide together how to tell the rest of your coworkers.

THINGS TO CONSIDER

PROS & CONS TO TELLING OTHERS BEFORE 2ND TRIMESTER:

- There is still the possibility of a miscarriage.
- It can be a way to put your support team in place.
- If you tell only some people early, you run the risk that they will tell others.
- It might be best to tell if you are terrible at keeping secrets.
- If you need some special considerations at work.
- If you have any medical concerns that would make it safer to share the news.

PROS & CONS OF TELLING OTHERS AFTER 2ND TRIMESTER:

- You may be showing, which can prompt people to ask.
- May depend on whether or not the pregnancy was planned.
- Can allow you and your partner to enjoy the time together.

IT'S A DATE
DETERMINING YOUR DUE DATE

Determining your due date requires that you know the exact day you ovulated or conceived, which can be a bit difficult to pinpoint.

However, most women do know the date they began their last period. That is why the date of your last period is used to determine your due date and how far along your pregnancy is.

HOW IS IT DONE?

For Traditional Pregnancy (Intercourse):
Uses the date you began your last period.
For women who have irregular periods, ultrasound may be the only way to determine the date of pregnancy.

IVF Pregnancy (In Vitro Fertilization):
The process whereby an egg is fertilized by sperm in a test tube or outside the body, which is then implanted into a person's uterus.

METHOD #1 (INTERCOURSE)

Determine the first day of your last period
Last Menstrual Period (LMP)

ADD

280 DAYS

=

Your Due Date

EXAMPLE BELOW

July 1st
First day of last period

+

280 DAYS

=

Due Date
April 7th

METHOD #2 (INTERCOURSE)

STEP 1
Determine the first day of your last period

Last Menstrual Period (LMP)

STEP 2
count back

3

months

STEP 3
add

1 + 7

year   days

=

Your Due Date

········· FOR EXAMPLE ·········

July 1st
THIS YEAR

April 1st
THIS YEAR

April 8th
NEXT YEAR

=

Due Date
April 8th

This method is based on a 28-day menstrual cycle, so dates may need to be adjusted for a shorter or longer cycle.

(IVF)

For a Fresh Transfer, Date of Extraction, or Fertilization   **ADD**   **266** DAYS   =   **Your Due Date**

3-Day-Old Embryos Transfer Date   **ADD**   **263** DAYS   =   **Your Due Date**

5-Day-Old Embryos Transfer Date   **ADD**   **261** DAYS   =   **Your Due Date**

THE SUPER EASY WAY TO CALCULATE YOUR DUE DATE
There are lots of online apps that can calculate your due date in seconds.

PICKING THE TEAM

CHOOSING YOUR PRACTITIONER

Now that you are pregnant, you'll need to select your team of medical professionals. In order for you to decide, you need to understand what each of them does.

OVERVIEW

Several factors will influence your decision; for example:

- Whether you or your baby have any complications, including conditions like diabetes, high blood pressure, or if you are overweight or having more than one baby.
- Where you want to give birth: in a hospital, birthing center, or at home.
- Whether you want a natural childbirth (unmedicated delivery).
- The type of pain management you want during labor and delivery.

TYPES OF BIRTH PRACTITIONERS

OBSTETRICIAN-GYNECOLOGIST · (OB-GYN)

A medical doctor who specializes in all aspects of pregnancy, from prenatal to postnatal care. They can provide medical and surgical care, deliver babies, and approve fertility treatments.

For high-risk pregnancies, or instances where a great degree of care is needed, an OB-GYN may be necessary.

FAMILY PRACTITIONER (FP)

A medical doctor who specializes in care of the whole family. Some FPs provide basic OB-GYN care but will refer you to an OB-GYN in high-risk cases.

CERTIFIED NURSE MIDWIFE (CNM)

Specially trained, licensed professionals who partner with pregnant individuals. They provide health services to those with low-risk pregnancies. Midwives are registered nurses with a master's degree in nursing, who focus on assisting childbirth.

Midwives work with obstetricians who are available in case of complications during pregnancy, labor, or delivery.

OTHER PRACTITIONERS

PERINATOLOGIST

Maternal-fetal medicine specialists, who focus on caring for pregnancies where there are special problems, such as:

· Diabetes · High Blood Pressure · Genetic Disorders · Other High Risks

DOULA

A doula specializes in helping families throughout pregnancy. They provide a support function, offering physical, emotional, and informational advice to women before, during, and after pregnancy. They do not provide any clinical medical care.

They can help you find childbirth classes, learn birthing techniques, write a birth plan, and provide labor, nursing support, etc.

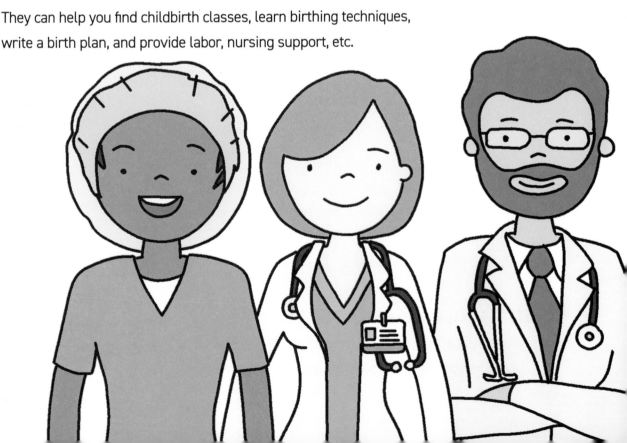

OBSTETRICIAN
FINDING A PREGNANCY DOCTOR

One of the first things you are going to want to do when trying to become or upon becoming pregnant is find an obstetrician. Here are some essential things you need to know.

OBSTETRICIAN-GYNECOLOGIST · (OB-GYN)

A medical doctor who specializes in all aspects of pregnancy from prenatal, labor, and delivery to some postpartum care. They can provide medical and surgical care for labor and delivery, as well as some fertility treatments. They also have training in gynecology (a physician who specializes in female reproductive health).

They will:

- Provide prenatal screenings, tests, and exams.
- Identify if there are any complications.
- Perform ultrasounds.
- Treat any health conditions.
- Manage labor and delivery—vaginal or C-section.
- Provide postpartum care.
- Monitor your baby's progress, size, weight and position.

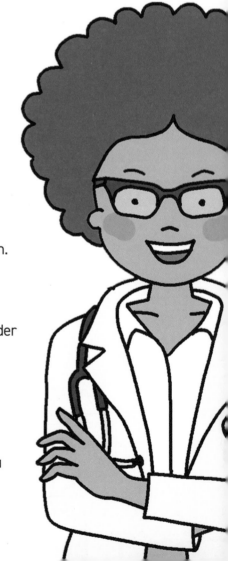

HOW TO FIND ONE?

- Get recommendations from your health-care/insurance provider to find someone who is covered by your plan.
- Talk to friends and relatives.

WHEN SHOULD YOU SEE THEM?

For regularly scheduled prenatal appointments or if you experience any problems during your pregnancy.

ARE THEY COVERED BY INSURANCE?

It is important to know if your doctor is in your insurer's network of coverage.

WHERE IS THEIR OFFICE LOCATED?

Is the doctor's office close to your home or workplace, and are the office hours compatible with your schedule?

WHERE DO THEY DELIVER?

Are you comfortable with that hospital? Does this hospital have a newborn intensive care unit (NICU)? What is the process if there are complications requiring a NICU?

DO YOUR EXPECTATIONS MATCH?

Does what is important to you match the potential doctor's priorities, and is their approach and level of care what you are looking for? Get their thoughts on medicated and unmedicated pain management, breastfeeding, and doulas and other support professionals, and review your birth plan with them to see that it matches what they can provide.

DO YOU HAVE SPECIAL NEEDS?

Ask the doctor if they have experience with patients who have high blood pressure, heart disease, diabetes, preterm labor, and preeclampsia, and about their experience dealing with complications.

ARE YOU COMPATIBLE?

Are you looking for a male or female doctor?
Are you comfortable openly discussing your body and pregnancy with them?
Are the doctor's explanations clear? Is the doctor easy to talk to?
Is the doctor open to answering questions after hours?
Is the doctor genuinely interested in you and meeting your personal needs?

WILL THEY PERSONALLY DELIVERY YOUR BABY?

Every practice is different; some will deliver your baby, and in others, the doctor on call may be the one to deliver your baby, meaning you may have a different doctor during delivery.

DOULA
YOUR PERSONAL TRAINER FOR PREGNANCY

These birth companions are there to help you feel safe, supported, and comfortable throughout the delivery of your baby. If it works with your budget, a doula is a wonderful addition to your team.

WHAT IS A DOULA?

A doula is a trained professional who provides you with physical, emotional, and educational support before, during, and after pregnancy. They try to make the birthing and postpartum experience positive by providing continuous care and support to the birthing individual as well as the partner.

NOTE: Doulas do not deliver babies or provide any medical prenatal treatment.

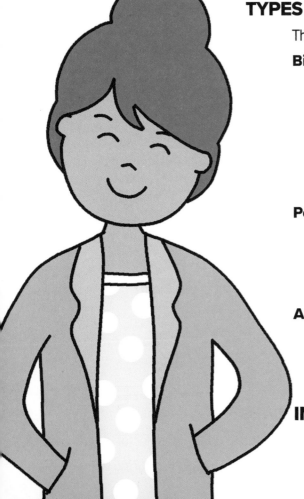

TYPES OF DOULAS

There are three types of doulas.

Birthing Doulas

Who support the birthing person and partner throughout the labor and delivery. They are trained to provide birthing support whether it is at home, a birthing center, or at a hospital.

Postpartum Doulas

Who support birth parents after the birth of their child, the postpartum period.

Antepartum Doulas

Who support those with high-risk pregnancies and on bed rest.

INSURANCE AND DOULAS

Not all health insurance plans cover the cost of a doula, so it is important to check with your provider.

WHAT A DOULA DOES

Doulas do different things depending on what you need, as well as their training.

Here is a list of the types of support a doula might provide:

- Childbirth education
- Answers to questions and information about the birthing process
- Prenatal massage and bodywork
- Relaxation therapy
- Explanations of procedures (keeps birthing couples informed)
- Emotional reassurance and encouragement
- Help in creating a calm, relaxed birthing environment
- Help communicating with medical staff
- Support and training for breastfeeding
- Pain management skills and techniques
- Help developing a birth plan
- Instructions on how to care for the baby

HOW TO FIND A DOULA

- Your doctor or health-care provider
- Friends and family
- Birthing-class instructor
- Your local hospital
- DONA International or CAPPA

INTERVIEWING A DOULA

Things to ask when interviewing a potential doula:

- What is their training/certification?
- How long have they been a doula, and how many births have they helped with?
- What is their philosophy on childbirth?
- What services and support do they provide?
- How to get in touch with them?
- How much do they charge?
- What is the typical process?

Remember, the doula is there to support you! So, you need to feel good and at ease with them. You should discuss all your needs and concerns.

MIDWIFE
ANOTHER ALTERNATIVE

If you have a healthy pregnancy, or are considering a home or natural birth, you might be interested in a midwife.

WHAT IS A MIDWIFE?

A midwife is a health-care professional who is trained to provide obstetric and gynecological care. Midwives can deliver babies at hospitals, clinics, birthing centers, or at home.

TYPES:

Certified Nurse Midwives (CNMs):

Have completed nursing school and have a graduate degree in midwifery.

Certified Midwives (CMs):

Have a master's degree in midwifery, but do not have a nursing school degree.

Certified Professional Midwives (CPMs):

Have completed coursework and are certified by North American Registry of Midwives.

Unlicensed or Lay Midwives:

Have some level of training and are certified or licensed to practice.

WHAT DO THEY DO?

Midwives provide:

- Pelvic exams
- Pap tests
- Birth control & family planning
- Postpartum care
- Breast exams
- Prenatal appointments
- Ultrasounds
- Prenatal blood work
- Lactation education
- STDs and STIs screening

WHAT DON'T THEY DO?

Midwives do not perform surgery and are not qualified to handle high-risk or complicated pregnancies.

WHY USE ONE?

Individuals may choose a midwife because they:

- Want a non-medicated birth.
- Want to give birth at home.

IS A MIDWIFE RIGHT FOR YOU?

If you have a healthy pregnancy with no complications, a midwife might be for you.

If you have conditions that raise the risk of complication, you will want to make sure your midwife is working closely with an OB or OB-GYN, or you may decide not to use a midwife.

Conditions that may lead to complications:

- High blood pressure
- A high-risk pregnancy
- Diabetes
- History of seizures
- Expecting multiples
- Requiring a C-section

QUESTIONS TO ASK A MIDWIFE:

- Where do you deliver babies?
- What local OB or OB-GYN do you work with?
- What insurance do you take?
- How long have you been a midwife?
- What kinds of tests and screenings do you perform?
- What is your process if there is an emergency?
- What kind of training do you have—CNM, CM, CPM, etc.?
- What is the total cost?
- What is your hospital transfer rate?
- Have you ever lost a baby?
- Do you have a support team?
- Do you offer postpartum care?
- Do you have any references?

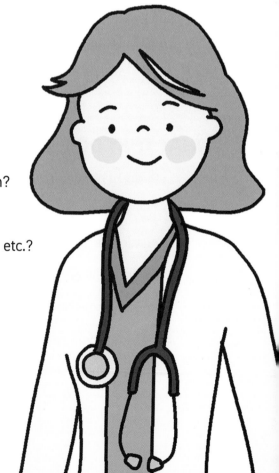

PEDIATRICIAN
FINDING A DOCTOR FOR BABY

Your baby's first examination may be with a hospital pediatrician or your chosen pediatrician. It depends on the hospital's policy and whether your newborn's outside doctor makes rounds there. If a hospital pediatrician checks your baby, those notes should be sent to your pediatrician.

WHAT IS A PEDIATRICIAN?

PEDIATRICIANS: Doctors who manage the health of infants, children, and adolescents. They treat everything ranging from minor illnesses to serious health concerns. Pediatricians also handle growth and development issues. They are the first person to call whenever your child is sick.

After you leave the hospital, your pediatrician will typically see your baby 48 to 72 hours later. They will see your child many times from birth to age two. Starting at ages two or three, your pediatrician will likely see your child once a year.

WHAT THEY DO:

- Perform physical exams.

- Track your baby's progress toward reaching developmental milestones.

- Administer vaccinations.

- Diagnose illnesses, infections, and injuries.

- Prescribe medications and treatments.

- Provide advice regarding your child's physical, emotional, and social development.

- Connect you with other pediatric specialists, if needed.

HOW TO FIND A PEDIATRICIAN

One of the biggest decisions you need to make before your baby arrives is selecting a pediatrician. It's important to have a pediatrician that you feel comfortable with before the baby is born, because, after your baby is born, you will be too busy to look for one.

WHEN LOOKING FOR A PEDIATRICIAN

1. Ask friends, family, and colleagues.

Start by asking your friends and family for their recommendations and compile a list.

2. Choose someone close to home.

You will want the office to be close to your home, as you will be going there a lot at first.

3. Check your insurance.

Check that the doctor is accepting new patients and takes your insurance.

4. Arrange a visit.

Once you have decided on a couple of doctors you like, you will want to schedule a meeting with the doctor and visit their office. Ask up front if there is any charge for this meeting.

5. Prepare questions.

When you meet with the pediatrician, you should be ready with a list of questions that pertain to you as well as topics of interest, like:

- How do you access the office after hours—phone, email, etc.?

- Circumcision vs. uncircumcised

- Vaccinations

- Board Certification

- Are they an AAP Member?

- Availability of lactation support

- Check the state's medical board website to see if there have been any complaints filed.

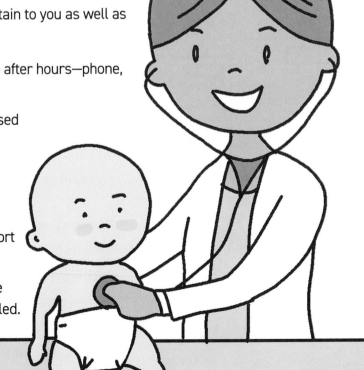

WHERE TO HAVE YOUR BABY

CHOOSING WHERE TO GIVE BIRTH

There are several options for giving birth, but determining where you want to give birth is influenced by several factors.

FACTORS TO CONSIDER

- Where your provider practices; not all doctors can deliver at any hospital.
- What your insurance will cover.
- If you have a high-risk pregnancy.
- If you are not planning a hospital birth, how close is it to a hospital?
- If a previous baby was delivered via a C-section.

WHAT ARE THE OPTIONS?

Hospitals

Hospitals provide the broadest range of medical professionals and emergency care, if needed. They have more options for pain management, including epidurals; operating rooms in case of emergencies; and some have a neonatal intensive care unit (NICU).

Traditional Hospital

You move from a labor/delivery room and then to a semiprivate room where your baby ideally will stay with you until you are released.

Family-Centered Care Hospital

Options for low-risk births include private rooms and baths (birthing suites) where you can labor, deliver, and recover all in one room. These rooms are decorated to feel more home like, but where medical staff is available. The baby stays with the birth parents most of the time.

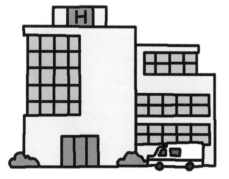

UNCOMPLICATED VAGINAL DELIVERY
YOU TYPICALLY GO HOME IN

1–2 DAYS

C-SECTION DELIVERY
YOU TYPICALLY GO HOME IN

3–4 DAYS

Birthing Center

Birth centers offer a more comfy, homelike setting with private rooms. Your family and friends can attend the birth. These centers typically have birthing tubs where you can relax during labor or have a water birth. They are usually located near a hospital; in case any complications arise, you are near a medical facility and staff.

If you are interested in giving birth at a center, you should go to one of their orientation sessions in order to check out the facility, meet the staff, ask questions, and learn about the center's policies. **NOTE:** Birthing centers do not provide anesthesia, so you will not have the option of an epidural or other pain-management medications. They also do not perform C-sections and do not handle preterm births.

Questions to ask:

- What is your hospital transfer rate?
- What events would require I be taken to the hospital?
- How is pain management handled?
- Is the center and staff state licensed?
- Who is the backup OB-GYN or doctor for the center?

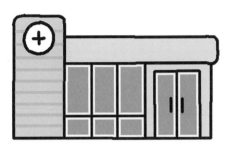

UNCOMPLICATED VAGINAL DELIVERY
YOU TYPICALLY GO HOME IN
4–6 HOURS
AND WILL BE VISITED BY A NURSE IN
72 HOURS

At-Home Birth

Home birth refers to delivering your baby in your own home. It's recommended that you only consider a home birth if you are healthy, you and your baby are free of any complications, you are not delivering multiples, and have not previously had a C-section.

If you choose to have a home birth, it is important to understand the risks and consult your health-care provider. Many people who have a home birth find it more relaxing and less stressful than in the hospital.

UNCOMPLICATED VAGINAL DELIVERY
YOU TYPICALLY
ARE HOME

MEDICAL HISTORY
LET'S GET PERSONAL

Now that you are pregnant, you are going to want to collect your family's medical history, and your partner's family's, for your health-care provider and your first prenatal visit.

WHY IT'S NEEDED

In order for your doctor to take the best care of you and assess your baby's risk of developing or inheriting diseases, your doctor is going to want specific details about both your family's and your partner's family's health history. This personal and medical history will help determine which prenatal tests and exams might be requested.

WHOSE INFO IS NEEDED?

The health history should include that of:

- The person whose egg was used.
- The person whose sperm fertilized the egg.
- Relatives.

WHAT KIND OF INFO IS NEEDED?

Family history of diseases, genetic disorders, or congenital malformations.
Listed below are some examples of what your doctor will want to know:

- Heart disease
- High blood pressure
- Stroke
- Cancer
- Diabetes
- Hemophilia
- Autism

- Parkinson's
- Osteoporosis
- Arthritis
- Alzheimer's disease
- Neural tube defect
- Muscular dystrophy
- Thyroid disorders

- Cystic fibrosis
- Cholesterol disease
- Tay-Sachs disease
- Multiple sclerosis
- Down syndrome
- Developmental disabilities
- Huntington's chorea

WHAT OTHER INFO IS NEEDED?

PERSONAL INFO:
- Age and ethnic group
- Any previous pregnancies
- Any delivery complications
- Mental health history
- Vaccinations
- Surgeries
- Allergies
- Asthma
- Gynecological history
- Medications taken

LIFESTYLE INFO:
- Sexual history
- Sexually transmitted diseases
- Drug use
- Alcohol use
- Tobacco use
- Exercise
- Nutrition/eating habits
- Vitamins/supplements

FAMILY HISTORY INFO:
- Gestational diabetes
- Preterm births

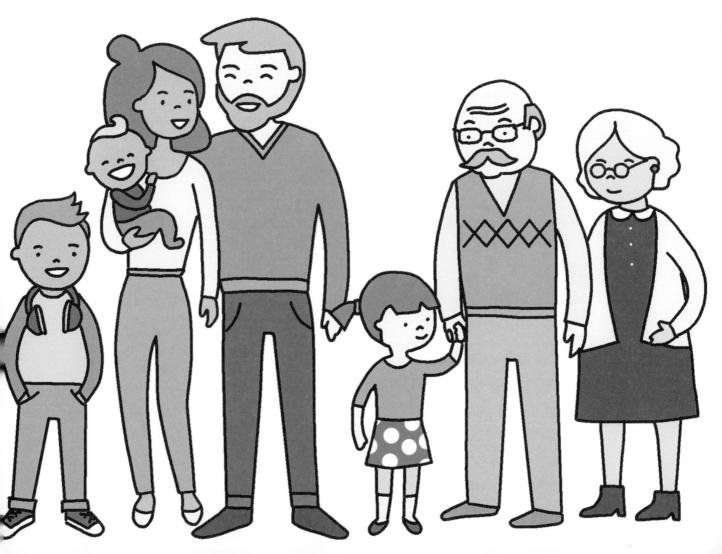

INSURANCE
THE BASICS

Figuring out medical insurance is a thrill for most people, which is why most of us hate it! Everyone's situation is different, but we try here to offer some guidance to help get you started.

WHAT INSURANCE?

Knowing what kind of coverage you and your partner have is the first place to start.

- None
- Employment-Based Insurance
- Affordable Care Act (ACA) Plans
- Medicaid
- Medicare
- State Insurance
- Direct Purchase Coverage

NO health insurance can deny you coverage just because you are pregnant.

QUALIFYING FOR INSURANCE

- You must enroll in a plan during the enrollment period, for both the employer or government marketplace plans.
- However, once you have given birth or adopted a child, you become eligible for coverage even if you are outside the enrollment period.
- If your income qualifies, you can enroll in Medicaid coverage at any time.

COVERAGE

- All health plans (except some older plans) cover certain preventive care with no out-of-pocket cost to you.

TYPICAL PRENATAL SERVICES COVERED:

- Testing and counseling for STDs
- RH incompatibility tests
- Folic acid supplements
- A range of prenatal tests
- Gestational diabetes tests
- Tobacco and drug cessation counseling
- Some labor and delivery costs
- Some hospital stay costs
- Breastfeeding counsel and equipment
- Birth control, after you deliver your baby

MOST-COMMON MATERNITY SERVICES COVERED:

Varies from plan to plan, but here are some areas of service you should look into to confirm if and how much your plan or prospective plan covers:

COVERAGE TO CHECK

- Labor and delivery services at a birthing center, home, or hospital
- Alternative birthing options
- High-risk pregnancies and complication coverage
- C-section coverage and recovery
- Lactation consultants
- Doula and midwife services
- Neonatal care
- Infertility treatment

QUESTIONS TO ASK

- Do we need to notify the insurance company when admitted to the hospital?
- What is my out-of-pocket cost (co-pay, coinsurance)?
- Is my obstetrician, hospital, and pediatrician in network?
- High-risk pregnancies and complication coverage?
- Are breast pumps and supplies covered?
- Is a miscarriage or termination if needed covered?
- Does my baby's cost count toward my deductible?
- How much is my deductible?
- Are childbirth classes covered?
- How long a hospital stay is covered?
- What are my maternity benefits?
- How much of my prenatal care is covered?
- Is my baby's stay in the hospital covered?
- Are water births covered?
- Is circumcision covered?

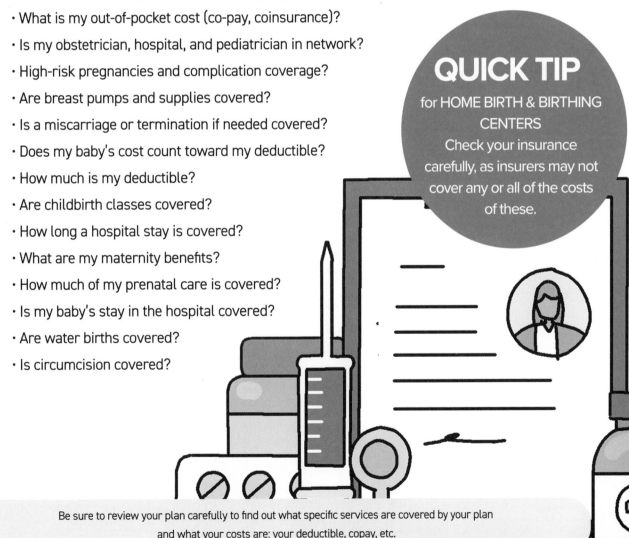

QUICK TIP
for HOME BIRTH & BIRTHING CENTERS
Check your insurance carefully, as insurers may not cover any or all of the costs of these.

Be sure to review your plan carefully to find out what specific services are covered by your plan and what your costs are: your deductible, copay, etc.

$$$WOW

BABIES ARE EXPENSIVE!

Here are some things to consider before your bundle of joy comes home.

THE AVERAGE MIDDLE-CLASS FAMILY'S YEARLY
SPENDING ON BABY IS BETWEEN

$12,000 and $14,000

WHAT TO LOOK INTO

GET INSURANCE

You just learned you are pregnant—it's time to check your health insurance or get some if you don't have any. You'll have to add your baby to the plan as soon as it is born.

REVIEW COVERAGE & COSTS

Find out what your insurance covers and what it doesn't. Look into the various out-of-pocket costs so you can plan for them.

EMPLOYER LEAVE POLICY

Understand what your employer's family leave policy is, what it covers, and for how long. If you don't have any paid leave, be sure to understand how much it will cost you to take off from work, and start saving now.

FINANCIAL AID

Research whether you qualify for any financial aid assistance.

LIFE INSURANCE

Consider getting life and/or disability insurance in case something happens to you.

BABY STUFF/GEAR

Start planning for the various costs you may incur after delivery, including:

- Diapers & wipes
- Child care
- Formula
- Clothing
- Stroller
- Bottles
- Toys
- Breastfeeding supplies
- Baby gear

ESTATE PLANNING

Update your wills, if you and your partner have them, to include your new baby. Make sure to add baby as a beneficiary to your insurance and retirement plans.

EDUCATION

Starting to save for your baby's education early can help in the long run. Consider investing in a 529 tax-advantaged college savings plan.

CREDIT CARD DEBT

Before baby arrives, it is a good idea to start cleaning up any high-balance credit card debt. If possible, pay it off; if not, try to cut back on spending until it is paid off. Also, look into transferring the debt to a lower-interest credit card.

TRACK YOUR SPENDING

If you don't have a budget and don't track your spending, it's time to do so. You will be surprised at all the little places where you might save money. Doing this will also help you understand your overall finances.

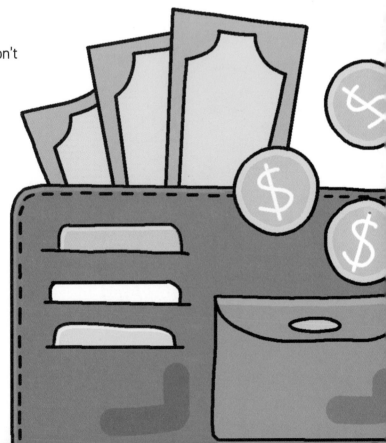

PEDIATRICIAN

Find a doctor you like in your insurance network. (**NOTE:** If your doctor is out of your network, consider one who is in instead; it will save you money.)

MATERNITY LEAVE

WHEN TO STOP WORKING

Choosing when to start maternity leave and how much time to take depends on your situation. Here are some things to consider in your decision-making process.

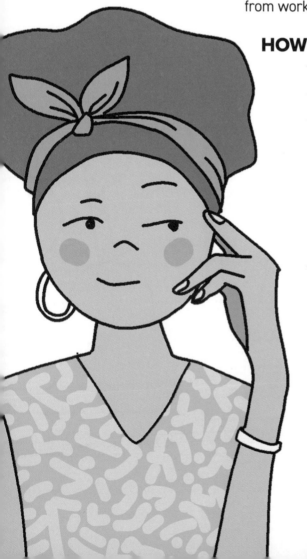

Mommy Hack

Speak with other women where you work who have taken maternity leave to get their thoughts on how they structured it and if they would have done anything differently.

WHAT IS IT?

MATERNITY LEAVE: The time Mom takes off from work following the birth or adoption of a child.

HOW LONG IS IT?

The time taken off could be anywhere from a few days to a year, depending on where you live and what benefits you have.

DO YOU STILL GET PAID?

This depends on where your live and your company's benefits.

WHAT IS IT FOR?

Maternity leave is intended to give the mother time to give birth, recover, and bond with her baby.

HOW DOES IT WORK?

There are several ways to structure the time off. In some cases, it might include a combination of:

- Government Benefits
- Paid Vacation Time
- Short-Term Disability
- Unpaid Time Off

STEPS FOR DECIDING ON LEAVE

1

UNDERSTAND YOUR OPTIONS

The first thing you are going to want to do is to find out what options are available to you. Do you qualify for government paid leave, short-term disability, paid, or unpaid time off? Explore what your company's policy is and what your insurance benefits for childbirth and time off are. It's also important to know your rights and the laws around maternity leave.

2

UNDERSTAND WHAT YOU CAN AFFORD

You will need to determine how long you can be off without pay or with only a portion of your salary.

3

SPEAK WITH YOUR CO-WORKERS

It can be helpful to speak with other co-workers who have taken time off for their pregnancy to get an idea about how it was structured and how they handled coming back to work.

4

TALK WITH YOUR EMPLOYER

Once you have some idea about the time you are interested in taking off, you can share it with your employer (your boss and human resources).

5

PAPERWORK

After speaking with your employer and your insurance company, fill out any required paperwork.

6

MAKE A PLAN

It is wise to work with your employer to create a plan for who and how your work will be handled while you are gone and how you will transition back after your maternity leave. This shows you are committed to your job and career.

7

WHEN TO START YOUR LEAVE

This will be different for each person depending on your financial needs, how much support you have, your pregnancy, benefits, and the type of work you do.

MATERNITY LEAVE

SPEAKING TO YOUR EMPLOYER

When deciding to take maternity leave, one thing you will need to do is talk to your employer. This is what you need to ask and know before you do.

QUICK TIP

Depending on the state that you live in, you may be entitled to additional benefits. Check your state's policies and laws regarding maternity leave.

FAMILY MEDICAL LEAVE ACT (FMLA)

Requires employers with 50 or more employees who live within 75 miles of their work to guarantee 12 weeks of unpaid leave without the employee losing their job or health benefits.

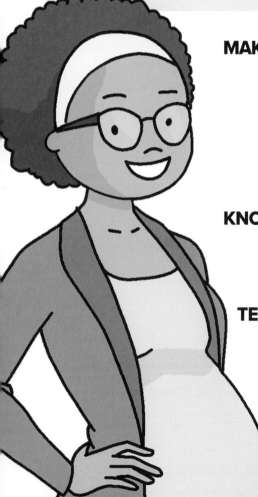

MAKE A PLAN

Determine how much time you want to take off as well as when you want to start and end your leave. Decide how accessible you want to be during your leave. For example, do you still want to work part-time, do you want a flexible schedule, and so on. Do you want to help figure out how your responsibilities are handled while on leave?

KNOW YOUR RIGHTS

Review your company's policies on pregnancy and maternity leave, and your rights according to Family Medical Leave Act (FMLA).

TELL YOUR EMPLOYER

When you are ready, set up a meeting with your manager to share the news and discuss your plans for maternity leave.

BE ORGANIZED

Document everything and keep all your maternity-related documents in a folder.

QUESTIONS FOR HUMAN RESOURCES

DOES THE COMPANY PAY FOR MATERNITY LEAVE?

Ask if you have maternity leave, and for how long, and if it is paid. Understanding what is covered and what is not is important because you may have to take time off without pay. How does the company's maternity leave work with the 12-week FMLA requirement?

DO YOU HAVE PAID TIME OFF (PTO)?

Does your company provide or allow the use of PTO (for doctors' appointments and other pregnancy-related absences)? PTO might be a combination of vacation, sick days, and personal days.

ARE THERE ANY RELATED BENEFITS?

Ask if there are any additional benefits, like a phased return, surrogacy assistance, and so on.

DUTIES AND ROLE?

Ask how the employer plans to handle your role while gone. Your job is protected under the Pregnancy Discrimination Act—you should understand the law and how it affects your job.

WHAT DO YOU NEED TO DO BEFORE TAKING LEAVE?

Understand what your company needs from you before you begin maternity leave.

WHAT PAPERWORK IS NEEDED?

Ask if there is any paperwork that needs to be completed or an agreement you need to sign. Take your time to review it carefully before signing.

WHAT ABOUT INSURANCE?

Find out how and when you can add your baby to your insurance and if there is additional cost.

WORKING REMOTELY?

Is your employer OK with you working remotely, and will they help set you up?

PATERNITY LEAVE

THINGS TO CONSIDER

What you need to know about paternity leave.

WHAT IS IT?

PATERNITY LEAVE: This is time granted to new fathers or partners who want to take off from work once a baby is born or a child is adopted or fostered.

WHAT'S IT FOR?

It gives the father or partner time to bond and provide child care for a new baby. It also can be a time for the father or partner to provide physical and emotional support to the birth mother.

HOW MUCH IS IT?

Generally, the benefit can be up to eight weeks with payment of as much as 60 to 70 percent of your normal wages. You will have had to work 5 to 18 months before being eligible for this benefit.

WHO IS ELIGIBLE?

Most states don't offer mandated paternity leave, and where it is offered, the benefits vary by state. There are currently only nine states and the District of Columbia who provide paid paternity leave.

- California
- Colorado
- Connecticut
- Washington, DC
- Massachusetts
- New Jersey
- New York
- Oregon
- Rhode Island
- Washington

Be sure to check your state's policies.

QUESTIONS TO ASK ABOUT PATERNITY

DOES THE COMPANY OFFER PATERNITY LEAVE?

Some employers refer to this as parental leave. Check with your company to find out what benefit, if any, they offer. Find out how much time your employer offers and when you can begin taking the time.

IS PATERNITY LEAVE PAID TIME OFF?

Most employers do not offer paid paternity leave, while others offer reduced pay or a combination.

DO I MEET THE COMPANY'S REQUIREMENTS?

If your company does offer paid leave, they may have specific qualification criteria that you will need to meet.

DO I HAVE TO TAKE THE LEAVE ALL AT ONCE?

Some companies give you the option of using the time all at once or taking the time within the 12 months following your baby's birth.

WHAT IS THE PROCESS FOR USING THE BENEFITS?

Some companies require that you use paternity leave only after first using other paid time or vacation days.

NOTICE FOR TAKING PATERNITY

Check what notification your employer requires before you begin taking paternity leave.

WORKING REMOTELY

Is your employer OK with remote work while on leave, and will they help set you up?

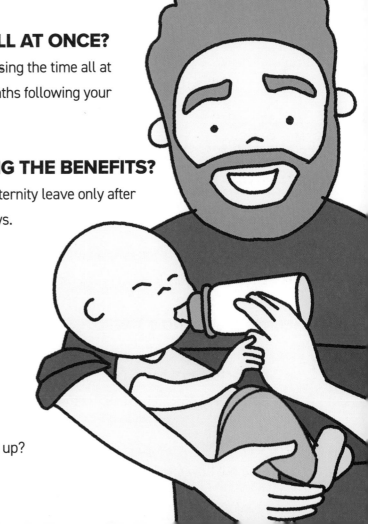

CHILD CARE
WHAT TO DO AND KNOW

The decision to start day care is one of the most difficult and stressful for any parent. Here are some things you need to know and some tips to help make the transition a bit less stressful.

Mommy Hack

As soon as you learn you are pregnant, you will need to determine if you will need child care. If you do, identifying where and applying early is important, as wait lists can be very long.

WHAT IS DAY CARE?

Day-care facilities come in two types:

1. GROUP DAY CARE

These facilities are similar to traditional schools and are state licensed. Children in day care vary in ages from infants to three-years-olds.

2. HOME DAY CARE

These facilities are run out of the provider's home. Some home day-care providers are accredited and have state licenses, but many are not.

2. NURSERY SCHOOL CO-OPS

Child-care centers that require parents participate in daily school duties.

TIPS FOR CHOOSING CHILD CARE

DO YOUR RESEARCH

Get recommendations from family, friends, other parents, your pediatrician, online, etc. Start looking early, as some might have a waiting list.

CHECK THE GROUND GAME

When you visit the facility, pay attention to the ratio of staff to children and how staff interacts with them. Babies need lots and lots of love and care for them to thrive. Caregivers should be down at the child's level, playing with or holding babies.

HYGIENE POLICY

Find out how often the toys, surfaces, and spaces are sanitized.

CHECK IT OUT

Visit the center yourself to assess whether it meets your needs. Look for:

- Current license
- Warm, friendly, and happy staff
- Clean environment
- Childproofed
- Stimulating daily activities
- Lots of age-appropriate books
- Lots of age-appropriate toys
- Shared space

MATCHING PHILOSOPHIES

Find out if you share the day care's parenting philosophy:

- Sick-child policy (What symptoms prevent attending?)
- Flexible drop-off and pickup times?
- Television (Is the TV on all day or used sparingly, if at all?)
- Discipline (Do the caregivers use time-outs, scoldings, etc.?)
- Food policy or plan (What snacks or drinks are provided?)
- Napping (When are naps? How are fussy babies put to sleep?)

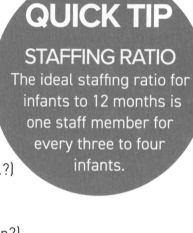

QUICK TIP

STAFFING RATIO
The ideal staffing ratio for infants to 12 months is one staff member for every three to four infants.

TALK, TALK, TALK

Make sure you communicate comfortably with the caregiver. In the morning, you should tell the caregiver how your little one slept the night before, if your child is teething, and whether your child ate breakfast. At the end of the day, you'll want to get similar information, such as the number of diapers used, when your child napped, and if your child seemed happy overall.

TRUST YOUR FEELINGS

If something feels wrong, keep searching. If something just doesn't feel right about the situation, investigate other options.

ADDRESS CONFLICT ASAP

If a conflict occurs, address issues right away; don't ignore them. Treat the caregiver with respect, but don't be afraid to speak up.

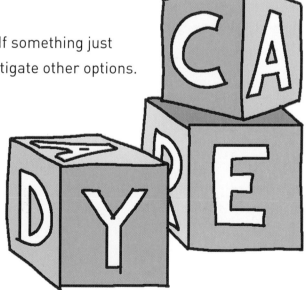

CHANGE UP

If things don't work out, make a switch.

MEDICATIONS

ARE MY DAILY MEDICATIONS OK?

Now that you are pregnant, you will need to be careful about any medication that you take.

OVERVIEW

It's generally recommended that you avoid taking any medications during pregnancy, especially during the first trimester.

Many individuals take medications on a regular basis due to health conditions, like diabetes, depression, or high blood pressure. If you have become pregnant or plan to become pregnant and are taking prescription medication, it's important to speak with your primary health-care provider to determine the risks and benefits of taking them while pregnant.

1. **Existing Prescriptions**

   Review all medications, prescription and nonprescription, and your medical history with your doctor to ensure your baby's and your safety.

2. **New Medications**

   Before taking any new medication or over-the-counter drugs, you should consult with your primary health-care provider or OB-GYN.

3. **Supplements**

   Don't take any vitamins or herbal supplements unless you have spoken to your doctor first.

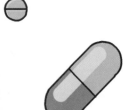

NOTE: The information provided is not a substitute for professional medical advice, diagnosis, or treatment. Always consult your obstetrician or primary health-care provider to ensure that a treatment or medication is right and safe for you and your baby.

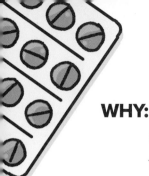

WHY:

Some medications, herbs, or supplements can cause problems for your baby; among them are:

- Birth Defects

- Premature Birth

- Low Birth Weight

- Neonatal Abstinence Syndrome (NAS)
  A condition where baby is exposed to drugs while in the womb, causing the baby to go through withdrawal after birth, which can lead to other serious complications.

- Miscarriage

- Stillbirth

CAUTION

Never take any medication while pregnant without first consulting your primary care provider or doctor to determine what is safe for you and your baby.

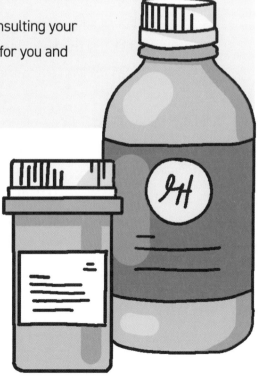

UPDATING WILL
GETTING YOUR AFFAIRS IN ORDER

Not what we want to think about, but if you have a will, it's a good time to update it, and, if you don't, consider getting one. These are the basic steps for putting a will together.

WHAT IS IT?

A will is a legal document that spells out your wishes regarding the care of your children, as well as the distribution of your assets after your death.

WHO NEEDS ONE?

Each individual parent should have one.

WHAT IS IN IT?

- It names the guardian of the child: the person or people who will raise your children when you are gone.
- It outlines the allocation of your assets: who gets what.
- It specifies who is the executor of the will: the person you have chosen to oversee the execution of your wishes.
- It outlines any trust arrangements.
- It outlines the kind of life-sustaining treatment you do and do not want to receive.

WHAT IS A TRUST?

This is a legal arrangement where a person or organization acts on behalf of another person. The trust holds the assets or property and distributes them according to your wishes. This saves time, reduces paperwork, and avoids fees and estate taxes. It can help you control when and how your assets are given to your children.

CHOOSING A GUARDIAN

GUARDIAN: The person or people to whom you have given the legal right to raise your kids should something happen to you.

This should be someone whom you trust to raise your children the way that you want them to be raised. You will want to speak to this person or people first to make sure they are willing to take on the responsibility.

WHO CAN CREATE A WILL?

- You
- A Lawyer
- A Trustee Corporation

NOTE: It is highly recommended that you use a lawyer to write your will, or at least have one take a look at what you have written yourself.

MAKING IT OFFICIAL

Once you have outlined your wishes, you then:

- Properly sign it.
- Have the signing witnessed by two adults. Witnesses should be someone other than your spouse, partner, or beneficiaries.

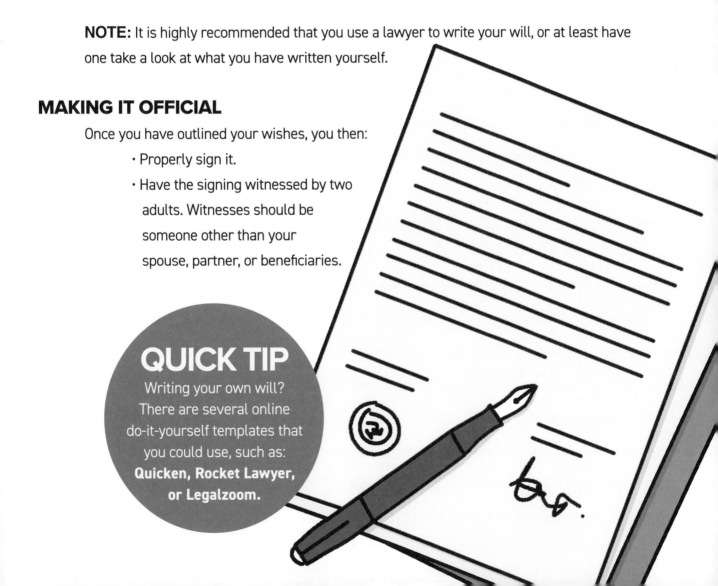

QUICK TIP

Writing your own will? There are several online do-it-yourself templates that you could use, such as: **Quicken, Rocket Lawyer, or Legalzoom.**

Eat well,
live well,
be well.

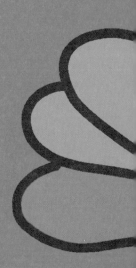

NUTRITION

Some healthy advice on what you need to know when you are eating for two.

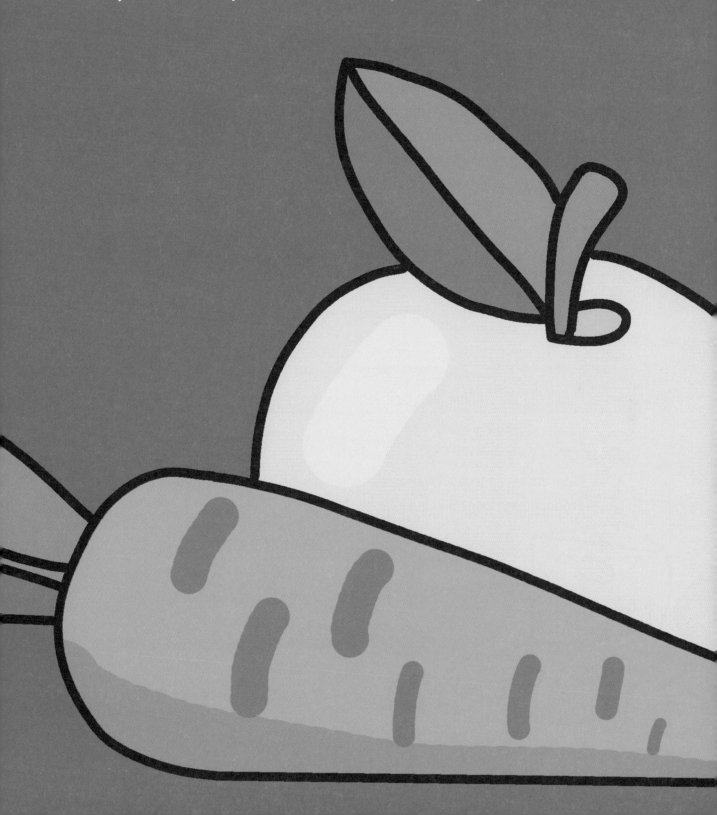

HEALTHY EATING
FOOD FOR THOUGHT

Good nutrition should be part of everyone's daily life, but when you are pregnant, it's even more important. Healthy choices help you have a healthy pregnancy and a healthy baby.

QUICK TIP

Eating healthy options can be challenging when you are nauseated with morning sickness. Taking a prenatal supplement can help ensure you get the needed vitamins and minerals.

WHY

You are no longer eating for you alone but for baby too. The development of a baby requires lots of important nutrients.

There are many important vitamins and minerals you should include in your diet.

TIPS FOR EATING HEALTHY

MIX IT UP

Eat a variety of fruits, vegetables, whole grains, fat-free or low-fat dairy products, and protein-rich foods.

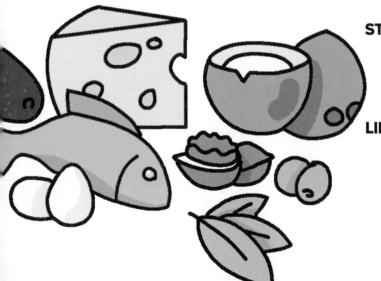

STEER CLEAR OF

Choose foods and beverages low in sugar, saturated fats, and salt.

LIMIT HIGHLY PROCESSED FOODS

Refined grains and starches like cookies, white bread, and snack foods are not healthy choices.

CHOOSE HEALTHY SNACKS

Try low-fat or fat-free yogurt with fruit, whole-grain crackers, low-fat cheeses, or vegetables with hummus.

EAT FISH

Try to eat 8 to 12 ounces (two to three times a week) of seafood that is high in healthy fats and low on mercury.

LAY OFF THE CAFFEINE

If you drink coffee or tea, choose decaffeinated with no sugar added. Pass on energy drinks.

STAY HYDRATED

Drinking lots of water during pregnancy is important. Stay away from drinks with added sugars, like soda, fruit drinks, and sports drinks.

LIMIT THE AMOUNT OF SUGARS

Use sugar in moderation—consult with your doctor on what is right for you.

CHOOSE FOOD HIGH IN FIBER

Try whole-grain breads, cereals, beans, rice, fruits, and vegetables.

PROTEIN

Eat protein like lean meats, chicken, and fish that are low in fat. Other healthy protein options are tofu, soy products, beans, nuts, and egg whites.

OILS

Use healthy, unsaturated oils like vegetable or olive oil.

VITAMINS AND MINERALS

Getting the right vitamins and minerals in your diet is important. Your doctor will more than likely recommend prenatal vitamins to ensure you do just that.

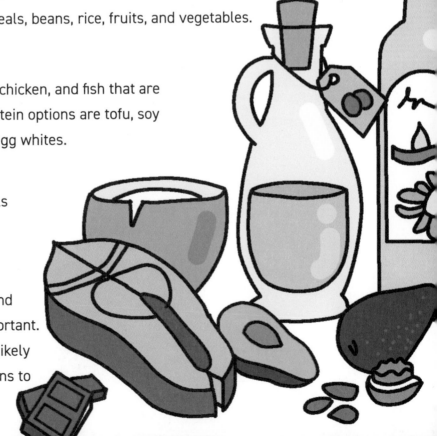

WEIGHT GAIN

HOW MUCH IS TOO MUCH?

Your weight gain during pregnancy is important to your baby and your health.

HOW MUCH WEIGHT SHOULD YOU GAIN?

Weight gain depends on a couple factors—it's primarily based on your body mass index (BMI) weight before pregnancy, but it is also based on your health and your baby's health.

WHAT IS BMI (Body Mass Index)?

The measure of body fat based on height and weight. This number is used to determine if a person is underweight, normal weight, or overweight.

TOO MUCH WEIGHT GAIN

Increases the risk of your baby being too large and you developing hypertension, gestational diabetes, delivery complications, and postpartum weight retention.

TOO LITTLE WEIGHT GAIN

Increases the risk of your baby being too small and other complications.

CDC Website: Centers for Disease Control and Prevention (CDC), Adult BMI Calculator

GOV Website: National Heart, Lung, and Blood Institute BMI Calculator

THE AVERAGE CALORIES NEEDED AND WEIGHT GAIN PER TRIMESTER

1ST TRIMESTER	2ND TRIMESTER	3RD TRIMESTER
1,800 Calories	**2,200 Calories**	**2,400 Calories**
PER DAY	PER DAY	PER DAY
2–4 Pounds	**12–14 Pounds**	**8–10 Pounds**
WEIGHT GAIN OVER 3 MONTHS	WEIGHT GAIN OVER 3 MONTHS	WEIGHT GAIN OVER 3 MONTHS

GENERAL GUIDELINES ON WEIGHT GAIN

Pre-Pregnancy Weight	Weight Gain (One Baby)	Weight Gain (Twins)
Underweight (BMI under 18.5)	28 to 40 lbs. (13 to 18 kg)	45 to 55 lbs. (22 to 28 kg)
Normal Weight (BMI 18.5 to 24.9)	25 to 35 lbs. (11 to 16 kg)	37 to 54 lbs. (17 to 25 kg)
Overweight (BMI 25 to 29.9)	15 to 25 lbs. (7 to 11 kg)	31 to 50 lbs. (14 to 23 kg)
Obesity (BMI 30 or more)	11 to 20 lbs. (5 to 9 kg)	25 to 42 lbs. (11 to 19 kg)

NOTE: Speak with your doctor to confirm the correct weight for you.

WHERE THE WEIGHT GOES (One Baby)

THE AVERAGE WEIGHT GAINS AND WHERE IT MAY GO

BABY: 7–8 lbs. (3 to 3.6 kg)

BREAST: 1–2 lbs. (0.5 to 1.4 kg)

UTERUS: 2 lbs. (0.9 kg)

PLACENTA: 1 1/2 lbs. (0.7 kg)

AMNIOTIC FLUID: 2 lbs. (0.9 kg)

INCREASED BLOOD: 3–4 lbs. (1.4 to 1.8 kg)

INCREASED FLUIDS: 2–3 lbs. (0.9 to 1.4 kg)

EXTRA FAT: 6–8 lbs. (2.7 to 3.6 kg)

FACT

Most women will gain **25–35 Pounds** 11.5 to 16 Kilograms during pregnancy.

CRAVINGS
FOOD FOR THOUGHT

I am having the munchies for pickles, ice cream, and peanut butter.

PREGNANCY CRAVINGS

Pregnancy cravings are strong urges to eat certain foods that affect many women during pregnancy. Sometimes these cravings are for common foods, and at other times they are for unusual food combinations or types of food the woman would normally not eat.

PICA CRAVING

The rare craving to eat nonfood substances.

- Chalk
- Laundry Starch
- Dirt
- Charcoal
- Sand
- Toothpaste
- Coffee Grounds
- Baking Soda
- Burnt Matches
- Soap
- Clay

CAUTION: These items can pose a risk to you and your baby. If you find yourself craving any nonfood items, contact your doctor.

WHY CRAVINGS?

There is no agreed-upon or known reason for these cravings.

Nutritional Needs: Some believe they are due to the body's desire for certain vitamins and minerals; however, there is no evidence for this.

Hormonal Changes: Others speculate that they might be due to hormones affecting the way some foods taste and smell.

WHAT TO DO ABOUT IT?

It's normal and natural to have food cravings. Satisfying them is fine as long as you continue to eat a healthy diet overall, manage your weight gain, and don't eat any of the foods that are on the no-no list.

MOST COMMON CRAVINGS

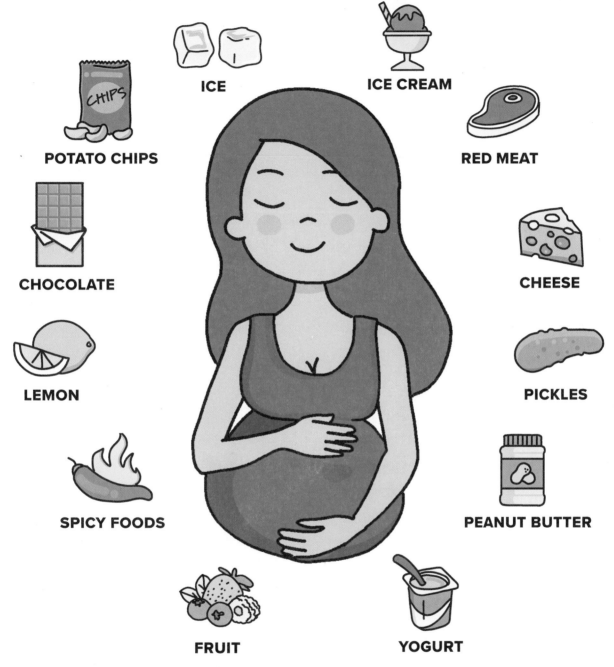

ICE

ICE CREAM

POTATO CHIPS

RED MEAT

CHOCOLATE

CHEESE

LEMON

PICKLES

SPICY FOODS

PEANUT BUTTER

FRUIT

YOGURT

PREGNANCY AVERSIONS

Pregnancy aversions are a strong revulsion to the taste and smell of certain foods during pregnancy. Food aversion during pregnancy is normal and common.

Common Food-Aversion Items:

· Eggs   · Onions   · Fish   · Seafood   · Garlic   · Meat   · Coffee

SUPPLEMENTS
PLUSING OUT YOUR DIET

Most doctors and midwives prescribe prenatal vitamins to fill any nutritional gaps, ensuring that you and your baby get the nourishment you need for a healthy pregnancy.

WHAT ARE PRENATAL VITAMINS?

Multi-vitamin supplements made for individuals who are pregnant or trying to become pregnant. They give your body the additional vitamins and minerals needed for pregnancy.

WHEN & WHY TO TAKE THEM?

They are meant to be taken before conception, during pregnancy, and while breastfeeding.

Before Conception:

Some birth defects happen very early in a pregnancy, before some women even know they are pregnant. It's recommended that you starting taking prenatal vitamins for three months before trying to get pregnant.

During Pregnancy:

With pregnancy comes an increased demand for vitamins and minerals. To meet that need, of course, a healthy diet is always best, but you may fall short of getting all the nutrients you and your baby need; prenatal vitamins help fill any gaps.

During Breastfeeding:

It's recommended that breastfeeding moms take some sort of multivitamin. You could continue taking your prenatal vitamin, but it contains more iron than is needed and might cause constipation. Speak to your doctor about what they recommend.

CAUTION: Consult your health-care provider or doctor before taking any medication or supplement to determine the amount that is safe and right for you and your baby.

NOTE: The information provided is not a substitute for professional medical advice, diagnosis, or treatment. Always consult your obstetrician or primary health-care provider to ensure that a treatment or medication is right for you and your child.

KEY VITAMINS CONTAINED

FOLIC ACID: 600 Micrograms

One of the most important vitamins, it promotes neural tube development and helps prevent birth defects of the brain and spinal cord.

CHOLINE: 450 Milligrams

Important for development of your baby's brain and spinal cord.

IODINE: 220 Milligrams

Critical for thyroid function and preventing miscarriage, stillbirth, stunted growth, mental disability, and deafness.

QUICK TIP

Prenatal vitamins should be taken as soon as you start trying to get pregnant—at least three months before becoming pregnant.

VITAMIN A: 770 Micrograms (2541 IU retinol activity equivalent)

Important for baby's eyes, bones, and central nervous system. Note that excessively high doses can lead to birth defects.

IRON: 27 Milligrams

Helps your body produce more red blood cells, which are necessary for oxygen and muscle and blood cell development in your baby.

DHA: 200 Milligrams

An omega-3 fatty acid that helps promote healthy eye and nervous system tissue development.

CALCIUM: 1000 Milligrams over 18
1300 Milligrams under 18

Important for Mom's and baby's bone health, and can help prevent preeclampsia and preterm birth.

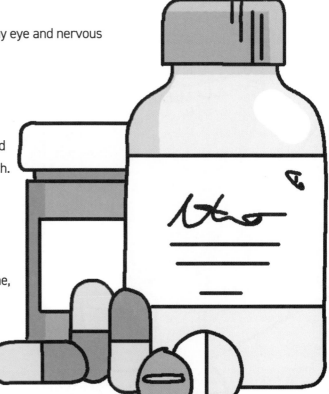

VITAMIN C: 80 Milligrams age 14–18
85 Milligrams age 19–50

Helps protect cells and has a role in the development of collagen, cartilage, tendons, bone, and skin.

VITAMIN D: 600 International Units

Promotes the development of healthy immune system and bones.

SUPPLEMENTS

I CAN'T STOMACH IT

Some women have a hard time taking prenatal vitamins; here are some tips that will help the medicine go down.

I CAN'T TAKE IT—WHY?

Some women struggle with taking prenatal vitamins for various reasons.

- Makes them nauseous.

- They have a hard time swallowing them.

- They make them constipated.

- They can't stand the taste of it when they burp.

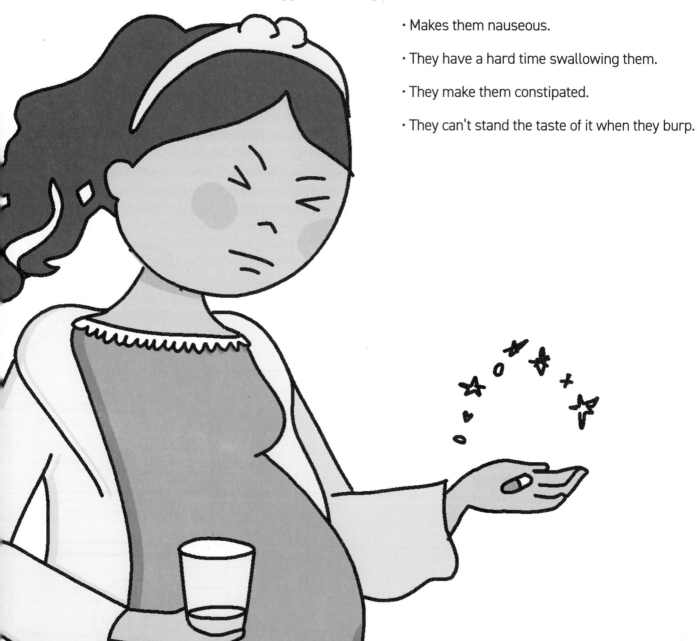

CUT IT UP

Try cutting the vitamin in half, and take half in the morning and half at night.

TAKE WITH FOOD

Never take a vitamin on empty stomach; that is one sure way to feel horrible. Try to take the pill after you have eaten.

LOOK FOR ANOTHER BRAND

It might be the brand and formulation that is causing the problem. Speak with your doctor to see if they can recommend another brand.

CHANGE TIMES

Try taking the pill at a time when you are least nauseous.

ASK YOUR DOCTOR

Share with your doctor any issue you may experience to get their recommendation.

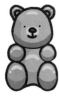

GUMMIES

Try a prenatal gummy. **NOTE:** You need to ensure that you are still getting the recommended daily allowance. Gummies may not contain iron, so if you are anemic, you may need an iron supplement.

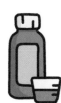

LIQUID VITAMINS

Look into a prenatal vitamin in liquid form. **NOTE:** You need to ensure that you are still getting the recommended daily allowance needed.

NO-NOS
FOODS TO AVOID

When they say watch what you eat, they are not kidding. Many foods and drinks can be dangerous when you are pregnant or breastfeeding.

QUICK TIP

If you are trying to get pregnant, **STOP** drinking alcohol! There is **NO** safe time for using alcohol during pregnancy, or while trying to get pregnant.

WHY CERTAIN FOODS?

1. Bacteria & Parasites: Contamination from viral bacteria or parasites are high in certain foods and can result in infections, such as:

Norovirus, Vibrio, E. coli, Salmonella, Toxoplasma, and Listeria.

2. Alcohol: Should absolutely be avoided, as it can cause very serious harm to your baby.

3. Heavy Metals: Certain foods contain high levels of mercury and other chemicals.

WHAT CAN HAPPEN?

They can cause serious health issues for your baby or result in life-threatening consequences like:

- Blindness
- Intellectual Disabilities
- Brain Damage
- Miscarriage
- Stillbirth
- Birth Defects
- Heart Defects
- Premature Birth
- Low Birth Weight

HOW DOES IT OCCUR?

Bacteria contamination can occur at any time during production, harvesting, processing, storage, transportation, or retailing.

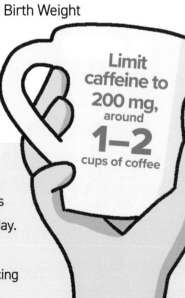

Limit caffeine to **200 mg**, around **1-2** cups of coffee

WHAT'S UP WITH CAFFEINE?

The American College of Obstetricians and Gynecologists (ACOG) recommends that pregnant individuals limit caffeine consumption to less than 200 mg per day.

WHY?

- It causes blood vessels in the uterus and placenta to constrict, reducing blood supply to the baby, reducing growth.
- It causes your blood pressure to go up.
- It dehydrates you.

FOODS TO AVOID OR BE CAREFUL WITH!

UNPASTEURIZED DAIRY:
Unpasteurized milks, butter, and creams have a high risk of bacterial contamination.

RAW OR UNDERCOOKED MEATS:
Meat patties, minced meat, pork, and poultry—cook thoroughly.

LUNCH/DELI MEAT:
Meat may become infected during processing and storage—cook throughly.

SUSHI: Avoid all raw fish, especially shellfish like oysters and clams.

RAW EGG PRODUCTS:
Like hollandaise sauce, homemade mayonnaise, salad dressing using raw eggs, ice cream, Bearnaise sauce, etc.

RAW SPROUTS:
Be careful with alfalfa, clover, radish, and mung bean sprouts, as they may contain salmonella—wash thoroughly.

CAFFEINE: Coffee, sodas, teas, and energy drinks should be avoided or limited to only 200 mg of caffeine per day.

RAW & UNDERCOOKED SEAFOOD: Also smoked fishes

RAW OR UNDERCOOKED EGGS:
Poached eggs, lightly cooked eggs, or salad dressing using uncooked eggs can be contaminated with salmonella bacteria.

HOT DOGS: Unless heated to steaming hot before being eaten.

ALCOHOL:
A definite no, and should be avoided.

UNPASTEURIZED JUICES:
Unpasteurized juices or freshly squeezed juices have a higher risk of bacterial contamination.

PATE AND MEAT SPREADS:
Have a high risk of bacterial infection.

UNPASTEURIZED CHEESE:
Avoid feta, brie, Camembert, blue-veined, and Mexican-style cheese for risk of bacterial contamination.

SEAFOOD TO AVOID!
DUE TO THEIR HIGHER LEVELS OF MERCURY

SHARK	**TUNA**	**ORANGE ROUGHY**
SWORDFISH	**MARLIN**	
KING MACKEREL	**TILEFISH**	

PREGNANCY SUPERFOODS

HERO FOODS

These powerful foods can help keep Mom and baby healthy throughout pregnancy.

WHAT IS A SUPERFOOD?

Foods that are nutrient dense and packed with vitamins, minerals, and antioxidants.

WHY ARE THEY IMPORTANT?

Adding superfoods to your diet helps improve your overall diet and health.

Vitamins and Minerals:

They are packed with healthy vitamins and minerals that the body needs.

Antioxidants and Flavonoids:

They contain molecules that help the body function more efficiently while protecting it from the damaging effects of toxins and stressors.

SUPERFOODS FOR PREGNANCY

EGGS

Thoroughly cooked eggs are a great source of protein, folate, iron, choline, and vitamins B12, A, E, and D.

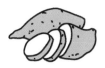

SWEET POTATOES

Full of nutritious fiber, vitamin B6, potassium, vitamin C, iron, copper, and beta-carotene.

BEANS AND LENTILS

Chickpeas, black beans, kidney beans, lentils, and soybeans are a great source of protein, iron, folate, fiber, calcium, and zinc.

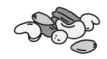

NUTS & SEEDS

Walnuts, almonds, pumpkin seeds, and sunflower seeds are full of healthy fats, omega-3, protein, magnesium, fiber, vitamin E, and minerals.

LEAN MEATS

Beef, turkey, chicken, and pork are great sources of protein and iron and full of B vitamins.

BANANAS

Good source of potassium and vitamins C and B6.

PLAIN YOGURT

Full of calcium, probiotics, and vitamin D.

Mommy Hack

Love your morning caffeine fix and socially drinking? Try decaffeinated coffee, and bring along some non-alcoholic beer when going to social events.

OATMEAL

Filled with fiber, protein, and vitamin B6.

GREEN VEGGIES

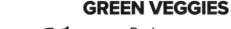
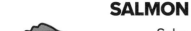

Dark-green veggies, spinach, asparagus, broccoli, brussels sprouts, and kale are great sources of antioxidants, calcium, potassium, fiber, folate, and vitamins A, C, and K.

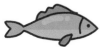

SALMON

Salmon, mackerel, and sardines are excellent sources of omega-3 (DHA & EPA), protein, iodine, and selenium.

BERRIES

Blackberries, blueberries, raspberries, and cranberries are a great source of protein, iron, folate, fiber, calcium, and zinc.

COTTAGE CHEESE

Full of calcium, protein, and iodine.

WHOLE GRAINS

Crackers, cereals, or breads are great sources of carbohydrates, zinc, iron, B vitamins, and fiber.

The journey
of a lifetime is
just beginning.

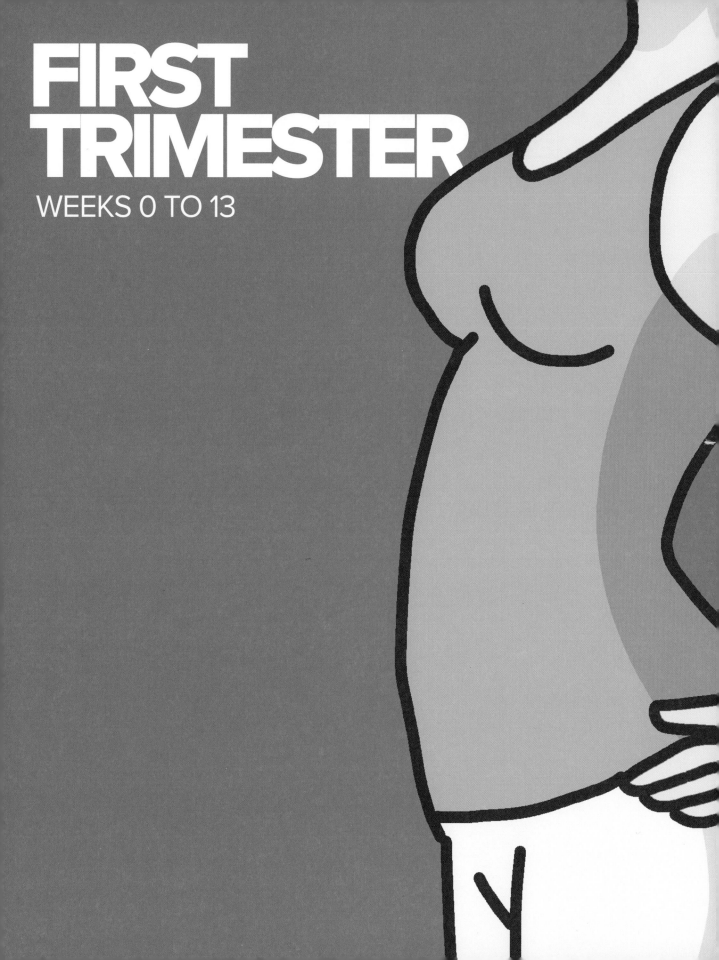

FIRST TRIMESTER

WEEKS 0 TO 13

YOUR BODY
1ST TRIMESTER: WEEKS 0–13

Welcome to the first phase of pregnancy: a lot is happening.

OVERVIEW

Your body is undergoing many changes as it prepares for pregnancy. Unfortunately, some of these changes come with a few less-than-thrilling symptoms.

Everyone experiences these symptoms differently. Some feel the symptoms more than others; some will glow with joy, while others feel completely miserable. Know that these symptoms usually ease up in the second trimester.

HOW LONG WILL IT LAST?

This phase begins at conception and lasts 13 weeks, or three months.

1st TRIMESTER (WEEKS 0–13)

YOUR HORMONES

To say that your hormones are running on overdrive is an understatement!

Several hormones are being produced that are driving many of the physical changes and symptoms you may be experiencing.

PHYSICAL CHANGES & SYMPTOMS

The typical changes and symptoms that begin in the first trimester:

- Tender, swollen, sore breasts
- Nausea or vomiting
- Increased urination
- Food cravings or aversions
- Cramping
- Skin changes
- Increased appetite
- Headaches

- Mood swings
- Spotting
- Weight changes
- Fatigue
- Spider veins
- Dizziness

- Heartburn
- Acne
- Constipation
- Bloating

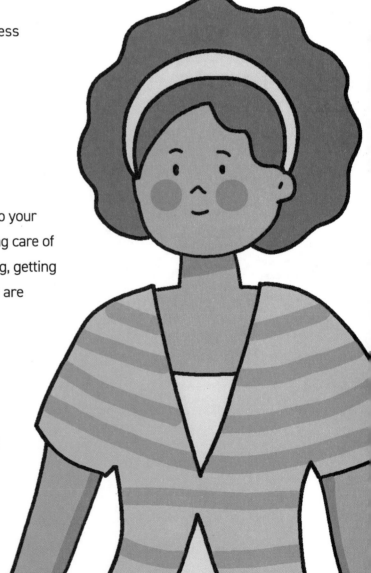

YOUR HEALTH

The first trimester brings lots of changes to your body and to your developing baby, so taking care of yourself is required. Eating right, exercising, getting enough rest, and taking a prenatal vitamin are very important.

MISCARRIAGE

A miscarriage can happen at any time in a pregnancy, but most happen in the first 12 weeks of a pregnancy, during the first trimester.

YOUR BABY
1ST TRIMESTER

What happens to your baby over the next three months.

OVERVIEW

This is a critical time for your baby, as it is growing faster than at any other time.

A lot happens in these three months, from rapidly dividing cells to implantation.

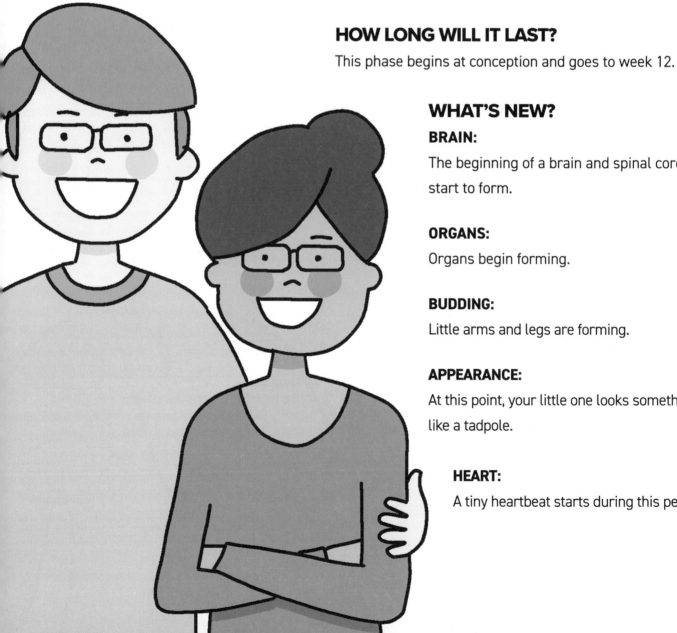

HOW LONG WILL IT LAST?

This phase begins at conception and goes to week 12.

WHAT'S NEW?

BRAIN:

The beginning of a brain and spinal cord start to form.

ORGANS:

Organs begin forming.

BUDDING:

Little arms and legs are forming.

APPEARANCE:

At this point, your little one looks something like a tadpole.

HEART:

A tiny heartbeat starts during this period.

WEEK	SIZE	WHAT IS HAPPENING
WK. 1	Nothing yet	You are actually not pregnant yet.
WK. 2	Nothing yet	Fertilization of your egg takes place near the end of this week.
WK. 3	The size of a pinhead	Sperm and egg fertilize in the fallopian tube to create a zygote; starts moving to the womb.
WK. 4	.04 in. Poppy Seed	The ball of cells implants in the lining of the uterus.
WK. 5	.10 in. Apple Seed	Hormones are on the rise. Your baby-to-be has a primitive circulatory system. The heart begins beating.
WK. 6	.25 in. Sweet Pea	Growth is rapid. The neural tube along the back from which the brain and spine will develop is closing.
WK. 7	0.333 in. Blueberry	Low limb buds are forming; they will become legs and arms.
WK. 8	0.6 in. Raspberry	Tiny nubs of fingers are forming, and eyes are becoming more apparent.
WK. 9	0.9 in. Grape	Arms continue to grow, and elbows form. Tiny toes are visible.
WK. 10	1.2 in. Peanut	Fingers and toes lose their webbing and lengthen. Tiny ears can be seen.
WK. 11	1.6 in. Fig	The baby is officially a fetus. Buds for future teeth begin to appear.
WK. 12	2.1 in. Plum	Fingernails are beginning to form. Intestines continue forming.
WK. 13	2.9 in. Lemon	Bones are beginning to form.

THE MUST-HAVES

FIRST TRIMESTER

Practical suggestions for common pregnancy issues.

GET THE RIGHT STUFF!

Scan the QR code to easily get our recommendations to start your pregnancy off on the right foot with the essentials you may need.

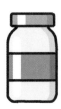

PRENATAL VITAMINS | SUPPLEMENTS

Folic acid, DHA, and iron are important components. You should also have a full range of vitamins and minerals, including calcium, vitamins D, C, A, E, Bs, zinc, and iodine. In addition, ask your doctor if taking an omega-3 supplement would be beneficial.

ANTACID

Look for an antacid that is calcium-carbonate based.

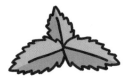

PEPPERMINT

Peppermint has been found by some to help soothe nausea. You can use peppermint tea (caffeine-free) or suck on peppermint candy.

GINGER

Ginger can have a calming effect on an upset stomach. There are ginger chews and capsules and ginger ale and ginger tea; you can also grate fresh ginger in warm water.

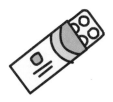

NAUSEA RELIEF

The American College of Obstetricians and Gynecologists (ACOG) recommends pyridoxine (vitamin B6) as a first choice. Some antihistamines, like doxylamine, can help. Speak to your doctor before taking any medication to make sure it is right for you and your baby.

STRETCH PANTS/LEGGINGS

Comfort is key, and having super-comfy stretch pants and leggings will go a long way to keeping you happy.

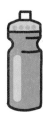

WATER BOTTLE

Staying hydrated is important, so having a BPA-free water bottle is great. Make sure it is one that will keep the water cool, as your temperature is going to be running high. Having a straw or top that you can drink directly out of is a plus.

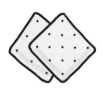

CRACKERS

This is a standard way to ease an upset stomach. Simple, plain crackers can also ease hunger pains. It might be wise to put some in your bag when you go out, and on your nightstand.

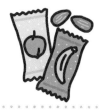

HEALTHY SNACKS

You will want to have lots of snacks handy; some good ones are protein bars, granola bars, and almonds.

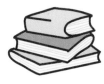

PREGNANCY INFO

Pregnancy is complicated, so getting the right information and knowledge is important. You can get that from books, videos, websites, blogs, and by taking pregnancy classes.

COMFY BRA

Your breasts are going to be tender; a soft and stretchy bra will be well worth the expense.

HORMONES
WHAT THE HELL IS GOING ON?

Hormones play a critical role in both preparing the body for birth and helping the baby develop; at the same time, they take expecting parents on a crazy roller-coaster ride.

WHAT ARE THEY & WHAT ARE THEY DOING?

HUMAN CHORIONIC GONADOTROPIN (hCG)

The hCG hormone is typically found in the body during pregnancy. It tells the body to start preparing for pregnancy. It's the hormone that home pregnancy tests look for to determine whether you are pregnant.

What hCG Does:

- hCG increases production of estrogen and progesterone.

hCG Side Effects:

- It is thought to cause morning sickness, nausea, and vomiting.

HUMAN PLACENTAL LACTOGEN (hPL)

What hPL Does:

- Provides nutrition to the fetus.

PROGESTERONE

What Progesterone Does:

- Prevents contraction of the uterus until delivery.
- Prepares the lining of the uterus for the egg.
- Prepares the breasts for producing milk.

Progesterone's Side Effects:

- Constipation
- Irritability and mood swings
- Acid reflux or heartburn
- Lowers blood pressure, resulting in dizziness.
- Gas
- Contributes to feelings of bloat and fatigue.

ESTROGEN

What Estrogen Does:

- Regulates the menstrual cycle.
- Prepares the breasts for producing milk.
- Helps the uterus grow.
- Helps the fetus grow and develop.
- Increased blood flow.

Estrogen's Side Effects:

- Achy and tender breasts
- Stuffy nose
- Glowing skin
- Increases urination
- Spider veins

RELAXIN

What Relaxin Does:

- Keeps the uterus relaxed during the first trimester.
- Helps with the growth of the placenta.
- Relaxes the body's ligaments.
- Softens and opens the cervix for delivery.
- Helps break your water during childbirth.

Relaxin Side Effects:

- Can make you a bit clumsy.

OXYTOCIN

Stimulates the pleasure centers of the brain and makes you feel great.

What Oxytocin Does:

- Gives you happy feelings.
- Starts the delivery contractions.
- Causes the uterus to contract.
- Stimulates bonding with baby while breastfeeding.

PROLACTIN

What Prolactin Does:

- Prepares the breasts for producing milk.

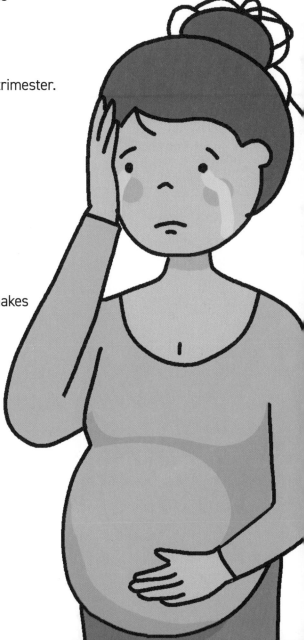

Fascinating Fact

The secretion of some of these hormones essentially turns off Mom's immune response, so it does not attack the baby.

MORNING SICKNESS

I'M SICK OF IT

Most women, around 70 percent, will experience morning sickness. It is one of the first signs of pregnancy.

QUICK TIP

Nausea tends to happen more often when the stomach is empty, so nibbling every couple of hours might help.

WHAT IS IT?

MORNING SICKNESS: The nausea and vomiting that occurs during pregnancy, which can be triggered by certain smells, foods, temperature, extra saliva, or without any trigger at all.

WHEN DOES IT BEGIN?

It typically starts around the sixth week of pregnancy and is at its worst during the ninth week.

WHEN DOES IT END?

Most women feel better by the second trimester, but, unfortunately, some will experience it throughout their pregnancy.

WHY DOES IT HAPPEN?

It's not known exactly why it happens, but it's thought to be connected to:

1. Hormonal Changes
2. Low Blood Sugar
3. Heightened sense of smell, which may lead you to find some food disgusting and others very attractive.
4. Stress and fatigue, which may worsen the condition.

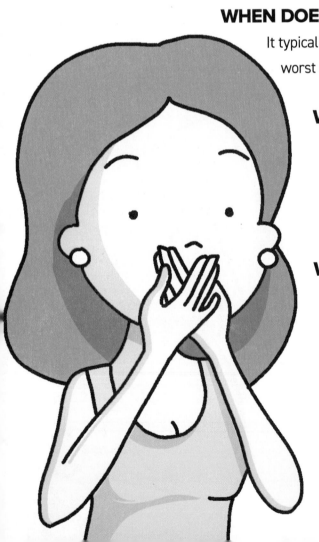

CAN IT HURT MY BABY?

Mild or moderate morning sickness has NOT been found to harm babies; however, you do want to make sure you stay hydrated and do not lose weight as a result of it.

TYPICAL MORNING SICKNESS

WHAT	WHEN	HOW OFTEN
Short spurts of feeling nauseated or vomiting.	Can happen at any time of day.	Can happen once or twice a day.

NOTE: Different people experience morning sickness differently and some not at all.

EXTREME MORNING SICKNESS

Called hyperemesis gravidarum, it can result in excessive nausea and vomiting. It can cause you to become dehydrated and lose weight.

HAPPENS MORE OFTEN IF A WOMAN:

- Is having her first baby.

- Is pregnant with a girl.

- Is pregnant with multiples.

- History of morning sickness runs in the family.

- Has a history of motion sickness or migraines.

- Is overweight.

- Has trophoblastic disease.

Mommy Hack

Have barf bags ready when you are out in case the unexpected happens. Colored bags are best, so you don't have to see it. Also have wipes or tissues available for clean up afterwards, and don't forget the mints!

If you experience extreme morning sickness, it is important to consult your health-care provider.

NOTE: The information provided is not a substitute for professional medical advice, diagnosis, or treatment. Always consult your obstetrician or primary health-care provider to ensure that a treatment or medication is right and safe for you and your baby.

MORNING SICKNESS

JUST MAKE IT STOP!

Morning sickness can be tough to manage, as what works for one person may not for another. Here are some tips for easing that queasy stomach.

Mommy Hack

Try keeping a small spray bottle of a fragrance that you like in your purse—that way, when you smell something awful, you can eliminate it with something you like.

TIPS FOR EASING MORNING SICKNESS

SNACK

Eating simple, bland snacks and munching between meals on yogurt, apple slices, cheese crackers, toast, or nuts may help settle your stomach. Pack snacks to take along when you leave home. Also, at night, keeping snacks at arm's reach can also help.

EAT MORE, BUT SMALLER MEALS

Nausea tends to happen when the stomach is empty or too full. So, try eating smaller meals more frequently (five to six meals throughout the day) to prevent your stomach becoming completely empty and not too full.

KEEP IT BLAND

Avoid fatty or spicy foods that might upset your stomach or are hard to digest. Try bananas, rice, potatoes, toast, broth, pretzels, or applesauce.

HYDRATE

Drink small amounts of fluid regularly throughout the day.

KEEP THE NOSE HAPPY

Avoid any odors and situations that may trigger nausea. The smell of lemons has been found by some to ease nausea. Find the scents that you like, and have them handy.

REST

Getting plenty of rest and reducing your stress levels may help reduce the nausea.

AIR IT OUT

Keep your spaces well ventilated; getting some fresh air or using a fan to circulate the air may help remove any odors that trigger it.

GINGER

Ginger is known to help ease nausea. Try ginger tea, ginger snaps, ginger ale, ginger biscuits, ginger tablets, or ginger candies.

PEPPERMINT

Peppermint-flavored candies may help relieve nausea.

ICE CUBES

If you are having a hard time keeping fluids down, try sucking on ice cubes.

ACUPRESSURE

Acupressure products put pressure on or stimulate certain points on your body to help relieve nausea; for example, a Sea-Band that exerts pressure on an acupressure point.

ACUPUNCTURE

The use of thin needles to stimulate and activate energy may relieve nausea.

MEDICATION

If you are having a hard time relieving morning sickness, consult your health-care provider about possible medications, Vitamin B6, doxylamine, or antiemetic drugs. They may also prescribe antihistamines, promethazine, metoclopramide, or an antacid.

PRENATAL VITAMINS

Taking prenatal vitamins with food or at night may help reduce nausea.

COLD MEALS

Some people find cold meals smell less and reduce their chances of nausea.

SPOTTING
WHAT'S IT ALL ABOUT?

Even light bleeding or a few drops of blood, called spotting, can be scary and can cause a lot of anxiety. However, spotting does not necessarily mean there is a problem.

WHAT IS IT?

SPOTTING:

It is light bleeding—a few drops of pink, red, or dark brown blood. It is lighter than your menstrual period and is common especially in the first trimester. The amount of blood wouldn't even cover a panty liner. It can happen at any time throughout pregnancy.

BLEEDING:

It is a heavier flow of blood than spotting. It will require a liner or pad to keep the blood from soaking through your clothes. It can happen at any time during one's pregnancy.

WARNING

Let your doctor know if you notice spotting or bleeding at any time during your pregnancy. Your provider will determine whether it is something serious and if it needs to be monitored.

CAUSES OF SPOTTING/BLEEDING

IMPLANTATION BLEEDING:

Implantation bleeding happens when the fertilized egg attaches itself to the lining of the uterus; it is a common cause of spotting early in a pregnancy. It can result in a couple of days of light bleeding and spotting.

CERVIX POLYP:

A harmless growth on the cervix, which is more likely to bleed during pregnancy due to increased levels of estrogen or an increase in the number of blood vessels in the tissue of the cervix due to pregnancy.

SEXUAL INTERCOURSE:

Sexual contact with the cervix during pregnancy could result in spotting or bleeding.

GYNECOLOGICAL EXAM:

Having an exam that comes in contact with the cervix might cause some spotting or bleeding.

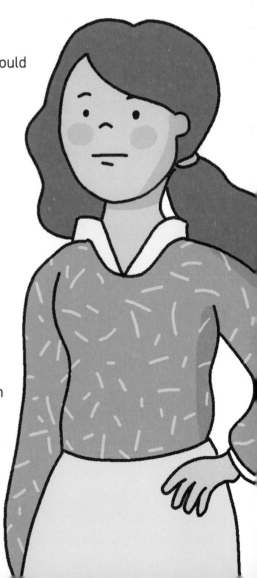

STRAINING:

Heavy lifting or intense exercise may cause bleeding or spotting.

ECTOPIC PREGNANCY:

A condition that occurs when the egg attaches itself outside of the uterus. This is a serious health concern for the mother.

MISCARRIAGE:

Occurs with brown or bright red bleeding, with or without cramps.

IMPLANTATION BLEEDING
THE WHAT, WHY, AND WHEN

WHAT IS IT?

IMPLANTATION BLEEDING/SPOTTING: It is a small amount of light spotting or bleeding—usually light pink or brown in color—it occurs in early pregnancy.

WHY DOES IT HAPPEN?

It's a result of the egg attaching itself to the lining of the uterus. It occurs in about 15 to 20 percent of women.

WHEN DOES IT HAPPEN?

It typically happens around 10 to 14 days after conception.

HOW LONG DOES IT LAST?

It can last a few hours to a couple of days.

WHEN TO CALL THE DOCTOR?

Always monitor any bleeding, taking note of the color, amount, and consistency because you will want to share this with your doctor.

If you experience heavy bleeding or clotting, let your health-care provider know right away, as it might be a sign of an early miscarriage.

IMPLANTATION BLEEDING VS. PERIOD
HOW TO TELL THE DIFFERENCE

Is it my period, or is it a symptom of pregnancy? Good question.
The symptoms for both are similar, but there are subtle differences.

	IMPLANTATION BLEEDING	NORMAL PMS/PERIOD
COLOR	Bleeding is light pink or brown.	Bleeding may start off pink and brown but changes to bright red.
FLOW	Generally light and spotty.	May start out light but progressively gets stronger.
DURATION	DAYS 1-2 — Light and short-lived, 1–3 days.	DAYS 4-7 — More intense and lasts longer, 4–7 days.
CRAMPING	Dull, mild cramping.	Moderate to severe cramping.
CLOTTING	Usually no clots.	It is normal to have some clotting.

HOW TO KNOW FOR SURE ONE WAY OR ANOTHER?

1. Your normal period arrives.   **2.** You have a positive pregnancy test.

PRENATAL VISITS

YOUR FIRST VISIT

Having good prenatal care is essential to your health and the health of your baby.

QUICK TIP

As soon as you think you are pregnant, and have confirmed it with a pregnancy test, you should make an appointment with your doctor.

WHAT IS IT?

PRENATAL VISITS: The regular appointments where your doctor, OB-GYN, or midwife examines you to make sure your pregnancy is going well and that your baby is healthy.

TYPICAL COMPLICATION-FREE PREGNANCY

PRENATAL VISIT SCHEDULE

FIRST PRENATAL VISIT: BETWEEN WEEKS 8 & 10

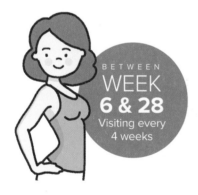

BETWEEN
WEEK
6 & 28
Visiting every
4 weeks

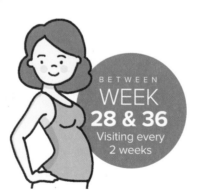

BETWEEN
WEEK
28 & 36
Visiting every
2 weeks

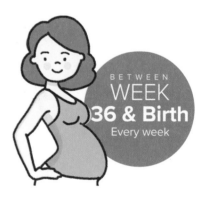

BETWEEN
WEEK
36 & Birth
Every week

MY FIRST VISIT—WHEN?

This appointment usually takes place somewhere between the eighth and tenth weeks of pregnancy.

WHAT DO I NEED?

You will need to have your medical history ready to share with your doctor.

Check out the medical history section, which includes all the things you'll need to pull together for your first prenatal visit.

FIRST PRENATAL VISIT: WHAT HAPPENS?

MEDICAL HISTORY
Your health-care provider will review your medical history.

PHYSICAL EXAM
There will be an overall physical to check your general health, including your weight, height, and blood pressure.

SYMPTOMS
You will be asked what pregnancy symptoms you are experiencing.

URINE TEST
A urine test will be done to check for kidney disease, bladder infection, bacteria, and your sugar and protein levels.

BLOOD TEST
For blood cell count, blood type, Rh status, iron levels (anemia), and infectious diseases like syphilis, HIV, and hepatitis, as well as your immunity to rubella and to screen for diseases like cystic fibrosis, diabetes, and thyroid dysfunction.

PRENATAL VITAMINS
Your doctor may prescribe prenatal vitamins or recommend a supplement with folic acid and iron.

VACCINATIONS
Discussing your vaccinations and if you are up to date or need any.

··· POSSIBLE ADDITIONAL TESTS ·····························
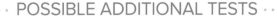

BREAST & PELVIC EXAM
To check the size and shape of the uterus.

PAP SMEAR
To check for cervical cancer.

ULTRASOUND
To view the baby's growth and position.

ULTRASOUND
LET'S TAKE A CLOSER LOOK

Your first ultrasound may be performed during the first trimester.

WHAT IS IT?

ULTRASOUND: A technique for creating images using sound waves. A wand that emits sound waves is placed on the pregnant person's belly. These sound waves bounce off the baby, creating images of it.

You may hear people use the term ultrasound or sonogram.
- Ultrasound: the device.
- Sonogram: the picture the ultrasound device creates.

WHEN SHOULD YOU HAVE IT?

Having your first ultrasound in the first trimester is becoming more common, but it is not standard practice for all doctors. You may have one done between weeks 10 and 12. However, depending on your doctor, it could be as early as seven weeks.

It is recommended that women get at least one ultrasound in the second trimester.

WHY HAVE IT?

- Confirms due date.
- Confirms viability of pregnancy.
- Checks for heartbeat.
- Checks fetal size.
- Checks if it's a multiple pregnancy.
- Checks for Down syndrome.

3D/4D ultrasounds are not standard care; optional if you want a closer look at baby.

3D Ultrasound

This type of ultrasound gives you a more dimensional image of your baby. The ideal time to get a 3D ultrasound is when your baby is between:

26 & 32 WEEKS

4D Ultrasound

This type of ultrasound is the same as 3D, but it also shows movement.

HOW IS IT DONE?

There are two methods that your first ultrasound might be performed.

1. Transabdominal Ultrasound

A wand, coated with a slippery gel, is run across your belly. It sends out sound waves that create an image of your baby.

2. Transvaginal Ultrasound

In order to get a closer look at your baby, a transvaginal ultrasound may be used, as your baby is soooooo small.

A wand, a little larger than a tampon, is gently inserted into your vagina that sends out sound waves to create an image of your baby. The wand does not reach the cervix and is safe for you and your baby.

TIME FOR YOUR CLOSE-UP

You may be asked to come to your ultrasound with a full bladder. This helps the ultrasound get a better picture, as it puts the baby in the perfect position for their pictures.

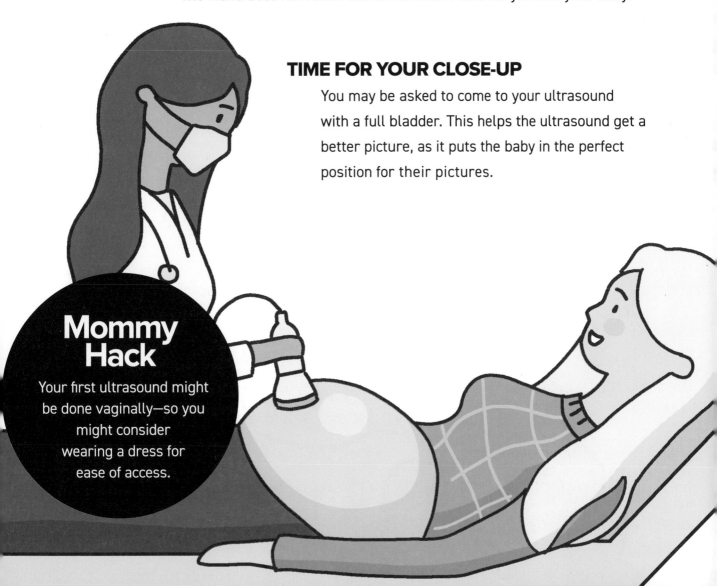

Mommy Hack

Your first ultrasound might be done vaginally—so you might consider wearing a dress for ease of access.

CONSTIPATION
THERE SEEMS TO BE A BACKUP

Constipation, unfortunately, is a common result of being pregnant.

WHAT IS IT?

CONSTIPATION: Means that you are struggling to poop, it is harder to go, or it happens less often than usual. Having less than three bowel movements a week is considered constipation. There may be abdominal discomfort as a result of infrequent bowel movements.

WHY?

Reasons for constipation:

1. Hormones

Oh, those hormones! The hormonal changes that are taking place that make being pregnant possible also can cause a bit of a backup. Progesterone, a hormone your body makes when pregnant, relaxes your intestines and bowels so that things slow down. Your bowels are not moving waste through as well as before. While this allows more time for your baby to absorb nutrients and water, it also makes poop harder to pass.

2. Your Baby

As it grows, more pressure is placed on the bowels, making it harder for excrement to move through and out.

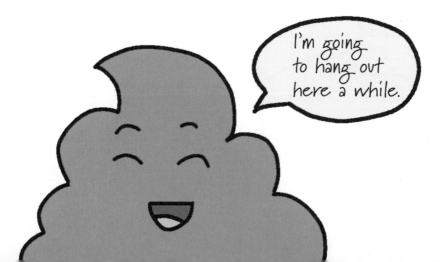

3. Iron

The iron in prenatal vitamins that is so important for pregnancy can also affect the breakdown of food, resulting in constipation.

4. Lifestyle

While pregnant, it's important to eat plenty of fiber, stay hydrated, and get enough exercise to help the digestive process.

WHEN?

You might begin to notice a difference in the second or third month of your pregnancy. Constipation can last all the way through birth and even a bit after.

TIPS FOR GETTING THINGS MOVING

 FIBER: Eat fiber-rich foods, fruits, grains, beans, peas, and lentils; aim for 25 g/day.

 HYDRATE: Drink 8 to 12 glasses of water a day, or try prune juice.

 ACTIVITY: Stay active; get regular exercise, like going on 10 to 15 minute walks or Kegel exercises.

 STOOL SOFTENERS: Speak with your doctor about a safe stool softener.

 SMALLER MEALS: Eat six smaller mini meals a day rather than three big ones.

 SUPPLEMENTS: Talk to your doctor about what fiber supplement they recommend.

 IRON: Consult your doctor about reducing the amount of iron supplement or if they recommend another option.

 PROBIOTICS: Eat foods with healthy bacteria, like yogurt, or ask your doctor about taking a probiotic supplement.

CAUTION
Do not take laxatives to treat constipation, as it might trigger contractions.

Speak with your doctor on the best treatment.

NOTE: The information provided is not a substitute for professional medical advice, diagnosis, or treatment. Always consult your obstetrician or primary health-care provider to ensure that a treatment or medication is right and safe for you and your baby.

HEADACHES
UGH, WHAT IS WITH THESE HEADACHES?

Headaches during pregnancy are common and can happen at any time throughout your pregnancy. They commonly happen during the first trimester.

WHAT IS IT?

HEADACHE: A pain in your head or face that can be either a dull constant pain or a throbbing pain.

CAUSES

There are different reasons why you might be having headaches:

- Hormones
- Hunger and low blood sugar
- Changes in your weight
- Posture
- Caffeine withdrawals
- Lack of sleep
- Certain foods
- Muscular strain
- High blood pressure
- Dehydration

TREATMENT & PREVENTION

- Avoid triggers
- Exercise regularly
- Eat regularly
- Get plenty of rest
- Practice relaxation techniques
- Limit stress
- Take medication
- Be sure you are not dehydrated

WHAT MEDICATION

Always contact your doctor before taking any medication, but Acetaminophen (Tylenol) may be recommended to treat headaches if natural treatments are not working.

CONCERNS

If you are having severe headaches after 20 weeks, with blurry vision, swelling, or pain in the abdomen, it might be due to other issues. Speak with your health-care provider to determine the right treatment.

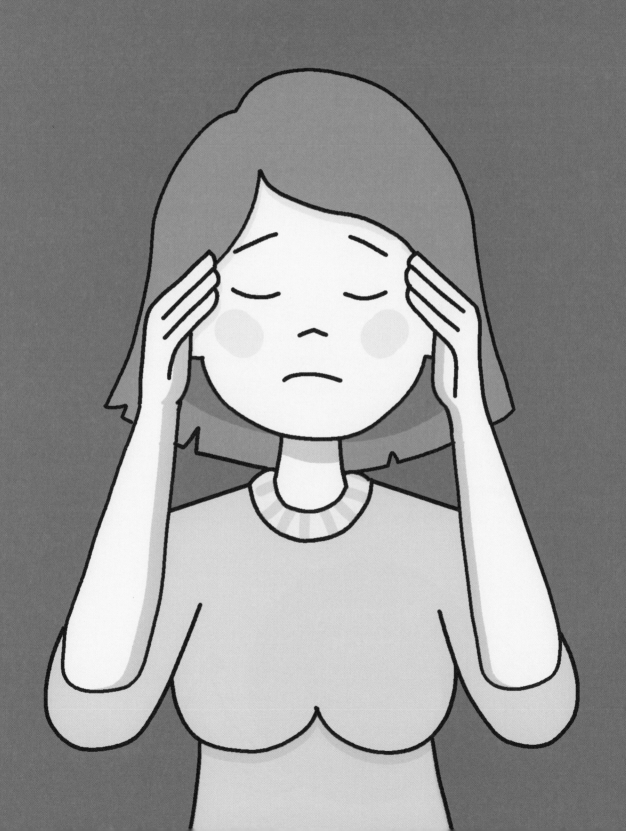

HEARTBURN
FEELING THE BURN

Another common symptom of pregnancy that affects half of all women is heartburn.

WHAT IS IT?

HEARTBURN: Also known as indigestion or acid reflux, is a burning irritation of the esophagus and stomach caused by stomach acid. The pain can be worse after eating or when you are lying down.

WHY IT HAPPENS?

Reasons for heartburn:

1. Hormones

The hormonal changes that occur during pregnancy cause the muscles that control the esophagus to relax, allowing acid to flow back up into the esophagus from the stomach.

2. Pressure from baby

Pressure on the stomach from the growing baby can cause reflux.

WHEN IT HAPPENS?

Heartburn can be felt in all three trimesters of your pregnancy. It usually is experienced soon after eating or drinking.

QUICK TIP

EASE THE BURN
Eating yogurt or drinking a glass of milk or almond milk can help ease heartburn. You can also try a bit of honey in a glass of warm milk.

Mommy Hack

Some fruits can help to reduce heartburn. Try: Papaya, Bananas, Watermelon, Apples, and Cantaloupe.

TIPS FOR EASING THE BURN

WATCH WHAT YOU EAT

Avoid fried, spicy, or fatty foods, as they can trigger heartburn—stick with bland foods.

LIMIT CAFFEINE & CHOCOLATE

Caffeine and chocolate, unfortunately, have been shown to trigger heartburn.

SPREAD OUT YOUR MEALS

Eat six smaller meals throughout the day instead of three large ones.

DRINK LIQUIDS

Drink less liquids with your meal but more throughout the day.

NO BEDTIME EATING

Don't eat late at night—give yourself three hours before going to bed after eating.

DON'T LIE DOWN

Wait one to two hours after eating before lying down to prevent acid reflux.

ELEVATE YOUR HEAD

Keep the head of your bed slightly elevated from the foot of the bed.

MEDICATIONS

Speak to your doctor about the best antacid for you or if they might prescribe any medication to ease the heartburn.

LIMIT CITRUS

Citrus products can cause heartburn; limit the amount consumed or water them down.

GUM

Chew on sugarless, mint-free gum half an hour after a meal.

PRENATAL EXERCISE

GETTING STARTED

Being physically active during pregnancy can be very healthy for you and your baby, but what exercises can you actually do?

WHAT IS IT?

PRENATAL EXERCISE: Mild-to-moderate exercise done during pregnancy to increase muscle tone, improve flexibility, and increase your positive self-image.

WHY DO IT?

Exercising while pregnant can reduce some of the negative side effects of pregnancy, and it also is believed to help prevent some serious complications.

- Improves circulation.
- Relieves back soreness.
- May result in an easier delivery.
- May reduce risk of gestational diabetes.
- Helps maintain healthy weight.
- Improves sleep.
- Reduces stress.
- Eases constipation.
- Reduces fatigue.
- Improves posture.

WHEN & HOW MUCH?

The American College of Obstetrics and Gynecology (ACOG) recommends a pregnant woman exercise 30 or more minutes per day, as long as you have no conditions that could make such activity risky.

RISKS

There are potential risks when exercising; be sure to consult your health-care provider to determine if and what type of exercise is right for you and your specific pregnancy. Moms should be careful of:

Overheating   Injury   Dehydration   Falling

SAFETY

Safety tips from the ACOG:

- Get clearance from your doctor to exercise.

- Drink plenty of water before, during, and after exercise.

- Wear support clothing, such as a sports bra or belly band.

- Don't become overheated, especially during the first trimester.

- Avoid lying flat on your back for too long, especially during the third trimester.

- Avoid contact sports and hot yoga.

- Wear loose-fitting clothing.

WHAT KINDS OF EXERCISE?

Exercise should be low impact and only mild to moderate in intensity.

EXERCISES

The possible types of exercise include:

Prenatal yoga

Low-impact aerobics

Stationary cycling

Light strength training

Walking

Swimming

QUICK TIP

Avoid any yoga poses that put pressure on the abdominal muscles, or involve twisting and putting pressure on your organs, especially in the later trimesters.

WARNING

Don't do any exercise program without first speaking with your health-care provider to ensure that it is right for you, your baby, and your specific pregnancy.

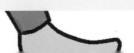

SPIDER VEINS

WHAT IS GOING ON?

Spider veins and varicose veins are another common, frustrating inconvenience during pregnancy.

WHAT ARE THEY?

Spider veins:

Existing small, red or bluish veins that have become swollen and thus are seen through the skin. They are typically seen on the legs but can occur anywhere on your body. They look a little like the threads of a spider's web.

Varicose veins:

Enlarged, squiggly, twisted veins that bulge out on the skin's surface. They can appear on the legs, ankles, feet, butt, and vaginal area.

Hemorrhoids:

A kind of varicose vein that develops in the anus or rectum.

WHY IS IT HAPPENING?

Hormonal Changes:

The increase of progestin can enlarge veins.

Increased Blood Volume:

Due to the increased volume of blood in pregnant women, the pressure on the blood vessels increases, causing the veins to swell.

Uterus Pressure:

Pressure from your growing baby also contributes to the development of spider and varicose veins.

Genetics:

If other family members had these, there is a strong possibility that you will too.

Straining:

Hemorrhoid can develop due to straining to poop when constipated.

TREATMENT

While It's not possible to completely prevent spider veins, varicose veins, or hemorrhoids, there are a few things you can do to minimize them.

- Watch your weight—stay within the recommend weight range.

- Sleep on your left side.

- Take your vitamins.

- Don't strain when going to the bathroom.

- Avoid sitting or standing for long periods.

- Exercise to increase your circulation by taking short walks.

- Wear compression socks or maturity stockings to increase circulation.

- Elevate your legs when sitting.

- Avoid tight or restrictive clothing—stick with loose, comfortable clothing.

- Avoid sitting with your legs crossed.

- After delivery, speak to your dermatologist about possible treatments.

- Take your vitamin C.

- Reduce your sodium intake.

- Drink plenty of water and eat high-fiber food to prevent constipation.

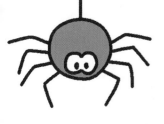

The good news is that spider veins and varicose veins that develop during pregnancy usually recede several weeks after delivery.

NOTE: The information provided is not a substitute for professional medical advice, diagnosis, or treatment. Always consult your obstetrician or primary health-care provider to ensure that a treatment or medication is right and safe for you and your baby.

INSOMNIA
I NEED TO SLEEP, I NEED TO SLEEP

One of the not-so-wonderful things that may occur during your pregnancy is "pregnancy insomnia." It is common and affects between 70 and 80 percent of moms.

WHAT IS IT?

PREGNANCY INSOMNIA: When you experience difficulty falling asleep or staying asleep, are waking up frequently, or a combination of all.

Mommy Hack

Some moms found sleep apps to be helpful to aid in falling and staying asleep. There are many available.

WHEN DOES IT HAPPEN?

Although it can occur at any time during pregnancy, it tends to happen in the first and third trimesters. Some people, unfortunately, experience insomnia throughout their entire pregnancy.

WHY DOES IT HAPPEN?

There are several factors that contribute to these restless nights.

- Hormones
- Heartburn
- Physical discomfort
- Restless leg syndrome
- Anxiety and worry
- Nausea
- Getting up frequently to pee
- Congestion

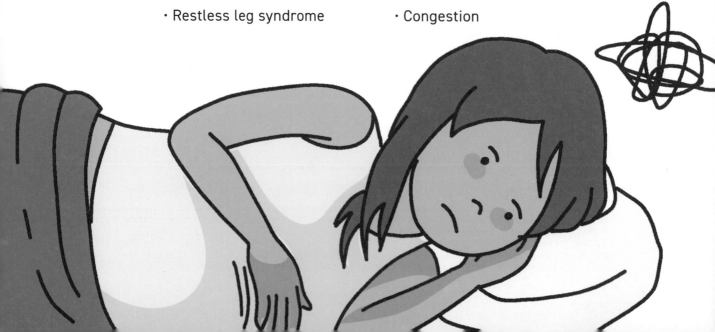

TIPS FOR GETTING ZZZs

BEDTIME ROUTINE

Go to bed and get up at the same time, avoid screen time an hour before bed, and make sure your bed is comfortable.

WATCH WHAT YOU EAT

Watch what you eat, and don't eat late at night; give yourself three hours before going to bed after eating to avoid triggering heartburn.

TRY DIFFERENT POSITIONS

Trying different sleeping positions may help to ease discomfort.

CALM YOUR MIND AND BODY

Prepare yourself for bed by calming your mind and relaxing your body.

CREATE THE RIGHT ENVIRONMENT

Make sure your room is at the right temperature for you. Make sure it is dark with no lights. Maybe play soothing music softly in the background.

TRY MEDITATION

Ease anxiety by mediating, or keep a journal next to your bed so that you can put down your thoughts and get them off your mind.

GET MOVING

Try getting a little regular physical activity during the day.

LIMIT NAP TIMES

During the day, make sure you don't take a very long nap, which might interfere with sleeping at night.

GET UP

If you can't get to sleep within 15 to 20 minutes, get up and find a boring activity, and do it for 15 minutes; then try to go back to sleep.

NASAL STRIPS

If congestion is preventing sleep, try using nasal strips and a humidifier.

ELECTRONIC DEVICES

Stop using electronic devices 30 minutes before going to bed.

1ST TRIMESTER CONCERNS

WHAT TO KNOW

The first trimester is one of the most critical for your baby, and, as a result, creates a lot of worry for parents. We have listed some of the more common symptoms to help you recognize issues and how to respond to them.

OVERVIEW

If a pregnancy is not viable, it will usually miscarry. This typically happens in the early weeks of pregnancy.

CONCERNS TO SHARE WITH THE DOCTOR

VAGINAL BLEEDING

While some spotting is normal, heavy bleeding can be a sign of miscarriage or ectopic pregnancy. If you experience heavy bleeding and cramps, it may indicate a potential miscarriage. It is important to see your doctor to get the proper treatment.

Ectopic pregnancy: When the fertilized egg implants outside of the uterus, you may experience heavy bleeding with sharp, lower abdominal pain and fever. This is an emergency and must be dealt with quickly.

EXCESSIVE NAUSEA & VOMITING

Some morning sickness is normal, but if it is severe, persistent, and making it hard to keep water down (dehydrating you), it is something to be concerned about. If this lasts more than 12 hours, call your doctor.

HIGH FEVER

If you experience a fever of 101°F or 38°C, it could be a sign of an underlying infection, which could affect your baby.

VAGINAL DISCHARGE & ITCHING

Some vaginal discharge is normal, unless it has an odor, is yellowish in color, or is accompanied by itching, which may indicate some other condition. See your doctor for the appropriate diagnosis and treatment.

PAIN & BURNING WHILE URINATING

This could be a sign of a bladder or urinary tract infection and can lead to serious illness, kidney infection, or preterm labor or birth, if left untreated.

LEG OR CALF PAIN AND SEVERE HEADACHE

Pain in the calf only on one side during the first trimester could be a sign of a developing blood clot. Consult your doctor.

ISSUES WITH CHRONIC DISEASES

Individuals with preexisting conditions, such as thyroid disease, diabetes, high blood pressure, asthma, or lupus should note any change in these conditions while pregnant.

DIZZINESS & SHORTNESS OF BREATH

If you are experiencing shortness of breath, a racing heart, or dizziness, you should contact your doctor and let them know.

CONTINUED WEIGHT LOSS

Tell your doctor of any weight loss.

NOTE: Always speak to your health-care provider should you experience any of the above symptoms.

I'm in love
with a human
I haven't met yet.

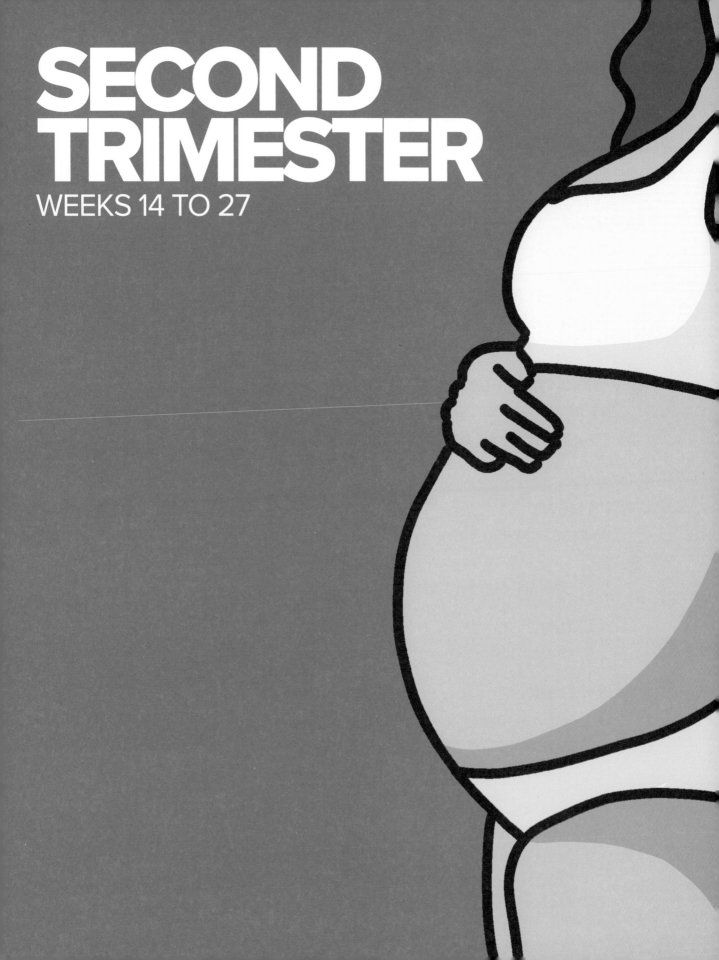

SECOND TRIMESTER

WEEKS 14 TO 27

YOUR BODY

2ND TRIMESTER: WEEKS 14 to 27

You made it through the first trimester—congrats!

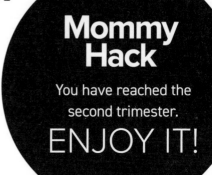

Mommy Hack

You have reached the second trimester. ENJOY IT!

OVERVIEW

Often this is the trimester when women feel their best during pregnancy. The nausea and vomiting may have eased up, if not completely stopped, and the risk of miscarriage has lessened.

HOW LONG WILL IT LAST?

This phase begins at week 14 and lasts until week 27 or three months.

2nd TRIMESTER (WEEKS 14 to 27)

WHAT'S NEW?

YOU ARE SHOWING NOW:

Your baby keeps growing and developing every day, and so do you! Your weight gain will increase in this trimester.

IT'S KICKING:

It's during this trimester that you will start to feel baby's first movements.

IN THE MOOD:

You may feel like you have more energy and are in a better mood because your hormones are leveling out. This is perfect timing since there is lot to do to prepare for baby.

THE BREASTS:

- They may not be as sore, but they are still growing.
- The skin and nipples may be darkening a bit.
- You might even begin to notice little bumps developing around the nipples; these glands produce an oily substance to keep the nipple from drying out.

SKIN:

- Your skin begins to stretch—the possible onset of stretch marks. These usually occur on the belly and breast.
- Your skin may become dry and itchy, especially on the belly.
- Your skin is more sensitive to the sun than before.
- A dark vertical line (linea nigra) appears down the middle of your belly, from navel to pubic area, which is completely normal.
- You may develop some dark patches on your face.

SWELLING:

You may find your ankles, hands, and face swelling a bit during this trimester.

ACHES & PAINS:

As you and your baby grow, you may begin to experience pain in your back. Your hormones are causing the ligaments of your hips and pelvis to relax, resulting in aches there.

TEETH:

You may notice that your teeth are somewhat loose, and your gums may bleed. This can happen because your hormones are affecting the ligaments and bones of your mouth.

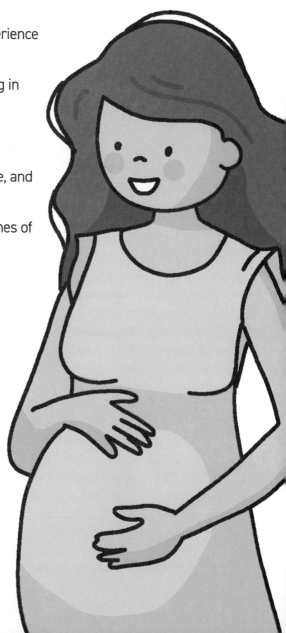

HEARTBURN:

Heartburn tends to worsen.

YOUR NOSE:

You may experience nasal congestion and nosebleeds due to increased blood flow.

(UTI) URINARY TRACT INFECTIONS:

UTIs are more likely during this trimester.

LEG PAIN:

You may be experiencing leg cramps, especially at night.

YOUR BABY
2ND TRIMESTER

The who, what, and when of the process of pregnancy.

OVERVIEW

The baby continues to grow and begins to look more like a little person.

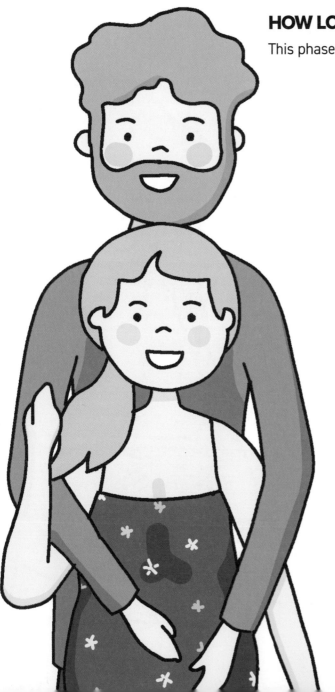

HOW LONG WILL IT LAST?

This phase begins at week 14 and goes to week 27.

WHAT'S NEW?

FINGERS & TOES:

Those tiny little fingers and toes are becoming more defined.

FACIAL FEATURES:

The eyelids, eyebrows, and eyelashes are developing.

EXPRESSIONS:

Your little one will be able to make faces—get your ultrasound pics ready!

MOVEMENT:

You may be feeling movement now, as baby will begin to stretch and even suck its thumb.

IT'S A . . . , IT'S A . . . ?

You will soon be able to tell if you are having a boy or girl; that is, if you want to know ahead of time.

WHAT DID YOU SAY?

During this time, your baby can also hear you.

WEEK	SIZE	WHAT IS HAPPENING
WK. 14	2.9 in. Lemon	Baby's skull and long bones are just beginning to harden.
WK. 15	3.4 in. Nectarine	Baby's sex may be able to be seen at this time.
WK. 16	4 in. Apple	Bones continue to develop and a scalp line/hair pattern is forming.
WK. 17	4.6 in. Avocado	Baby's head is erect now, skin is thickening, and its eyes can slowly move.
WK. 18	5.1 in. Pear	Toenails begin developing. Your baby is more active, rolling, and flipping.
WK. 19	5.6 in. Bell Pepper	Baby might begin to hear slightly. The baby's digestive system starts working.
WK. 20	6 in. Big Tomato	A coating called vernix caseosa is forming to protect baby's skin.
WK. 21	7.5 in. Artichoke	You might begin to feel baby's movements. Baby is sleeping and waking.
WK. 22	9 in. Carrot	Baby is developing the sucking reflex, enabling it to suck its thumb.
WK. 23	10.9 in. Mango	Eyebrows and hair are visible.
WK. 24	11.4 in. Grapefruit	Fingerprints and footprints are beginning to form.
WK. 25	11.8 in. Corn	Skin begins to wrinkle in places, and you might be able to see tiny capillaries.
WK. 26	13.6 in. Rutabaga	Baby might begin responding to familiar voices.
WK. 27	14 in. Lettuce	Nervous system continues to develop.

THE MUST-HAVES
2ND TRIMESTER

Practical suggestions for common pregnancy issues.

GET THE RIGHT STUFF!

Scan the QR code to easily get our recommendations for the essentials you may need for the second trimester.

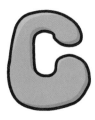

PREGNANCY PILLOW

The pillow should help support your spine, shoulders, belly, neck, knees, and ankles. They come in many shapes and sizes and styles from U-shaped and C-shaped to wedges. They can be filled with different materials: those with memory foam provide the most support, but some people find they sleep too warm. Whichever pillow you choose, it should have a cover that is easily removed for washing.

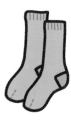

COMPRESSION SOCKS or HOSE

Make sure they provide a tight but comfortable fit. There are several styles, but the most effective are knee high or pantyhose. There are different levels of compression, depending on the amount of swelling you are experiencing. Speak to your doctor about the right level of compression for you.

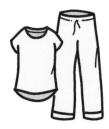

COMFY PJs

Having some super comfy sleepwear is a nice thing to have, as any little plea-sure is a gift. If you are planning to breastfeed, this is a great time to pick PJs up with buttons or an overlapping V in the neckline to allow for feeding later.

BODY/BELLY CREAM

As your belly bump grows, you will want to invest in some belly cream or butter to help avoid itching and discomfort; it may also help you avoid stretch marks.

BELLY BAND/PANTS EXTENDERS

These clever devices grow with you as you baby grows, allowing you to expand your current pants' and shorts' waists, so you can wear them a bit longer.

CONSTIPATION RELIEF

If constipation hasn't already kicked in, you may experience it soon. If or when it does, try the natural treatments, and if they don't work, speak to your doctor about the right treatment for you and your pregnancy.

BRA EXTENDERS

These inexpensive devices give you a little extra room for your growing breasts, which gives you a little extra time before you commit to a nursing bra.

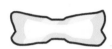

NASAL STRIPS

Nasal congestion will be starting and having something that makes breathing a bit easier might make sleeping a little easier too.

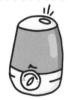

HUMIDIFIER

These can be helpful to loosen up congestion and help you breathe easier. Look for a cool-mist vaporizer or humidifier.

COMFY, SUPPORTIVE SHOES

There is nothing like a comfy pair of shoes when your feet start to swell and cramp. Look for slip-on flats with good support and padding. You might also consider a comfy pair of sandals.

HEARTBURN RELIEF

Although heartburn can happen in any trimester, the second is where most women begin to experience it. Speak to your doctor about the right medication for you and your baby.

MATERNITY CLOTHING

You are beginning to show; it's time to invest in some maternity clothing.

BACK PAIN
I NEED A LITTLE SUPPORT HERE

Back pain during pregnancy is extremely common. It may occur throughout your pregnancy, but in the second and, especially, third trimesters, those aches and pains can intensify.

WHAT CAUSES IT?

HORMONAL CHANGES:

During the first trimester, the levels of progesterone increase in the body, causing muscles and ligaments around the pelvis to relax. This loosening of the ligaments of the joints can cause back pain.

Another hormone called relaxin, released during the second trimester, also relaxes ligaments and joints in the pelvic area and affects the ligaments of the spine, causing a shift in posture and backaches.

STRESS:

Being pregnant can be stressful, and stress can have a physical impact, including stiffness and back pain.

POOR POSTURE:

In the second trimester, your baby is BIG, which changes your body's center of gravity and can cause you to lean back to balance the extra weight. This puts a strain on the back and can cause low-back pain.

WEIGHT:

Just adding 20 to 30 extra pounds is enough to put strain on your back, and it does.

WEAKENED ABDOMINAL MUSCLES:

There are two muscles that run along both sides of your abdomen. As your baby grows, these muscles stretch, becoming weaker and sometimes causing them to separate, resulting in back pain.

NOTE: The information provided is not a substitute for professional medical advice, diagnosis, or treatment. Always consult your obstetrician or primary health-care provider to ensure that a treatment or medication is right and safe for you and your baby.

TIPS FOR EASING BACK PAIN

MEDICATION:

Speak to your doctor about safe pain medication.

STRETCHING:

Regularly stretching the lower back and prenatal yoga are two ways to strengthen back muscles, as are other pregnancy-friendly exercises and swimming.

SIDE SLEEPING:

Sleeping on your side with a regular or pregnancy pillow between your legs and below your abdomen relieves backaches and pain.

WARM COMPRESSES:

Use a warm compress to relax tight muscles and reduce inflammation.

CHANGE POSTURE:

Change or correct your posture; stand and sit in an upright position.

MATERNITY BELT:

Get extra support by wearing a maternity belt.

LUMBAR PILLOW:

Use a lumbar pillow for extra back support while sitting.

PRENATAL MASSAGE:

Eases sore muscles, reduces stress, and increases range of motion.

KINESIOLOGY TAPE:

Kinesiology tape or spider tape can support your posture and ease aches and pains associated with a growing belly.

ACUPUNCTURE/CHIROPRACTOR/PHYSICAL THERAPY:

Use professionals who specialize in pregnancy back pain.

SUPPORTIVE FOOTWEAR:

No high heels! Wear flats or shoes with good arch support.

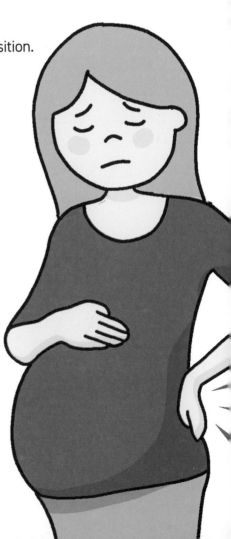

MAKING IT LAST
BELLY BANDS, BELT EXTENDERS, ETC.

What are all of these things, and what is their function?

5 FASHION HACKS

TO MAKE YOUR CLOTHES LAST LONGER

BELLY BANDS

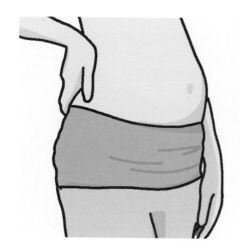

A flexible, tube-like garment that is worn around and over your pants and belly. As your bump grows, regular pants just won't close. The belly band hides the fact that your pants are not buttoned or zipped all the way up.

It is also a way to extend your wardrobe just a bit longer and can be worn as part of your outfit.
NOTE: Belly bands aren't meant for support.

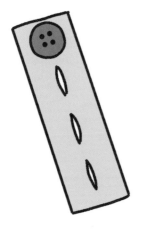

BELT EXTENDERS

These elastic waist extenders are designed with slots that fit over the button on your pants. The button on the extender goes into your pants' existing button hole. They can extend your pants between 1/2 to 2 1/2 inches.

They come in several styles and colors.

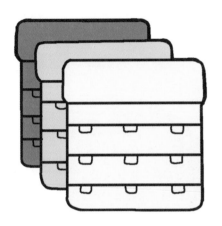

BRA EXTENDERS

Bra extenders attach to the back of your bra, giving you the extra room you will need as your breasts start growing; they're great for when you are not quite ready to commit to a new or nursing bra.

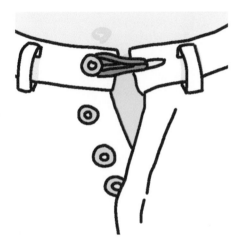

DIY PANTS EXTENDERS

If you don't want to buy a belt extender, here is a clever do-it-yourself trick:

Hook a rubber band or hair tie onto the button and loop it through the button hole and back over the button.

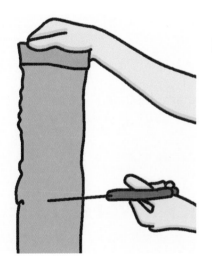

DIY BELLY BANDS

A clever idea for a homemade belly band is to take a pair of support hose and cut them above the crotch. You can slip this on just like a belly band and wear it under your shirt.

NOTE: It, too, won't give you the level of support that an actual belly band does.

LOOKING GOOD
MATERNITY LOOKS YOU WILL LIKE

Why can't I look good while pregnant? You can! Here are some ideas every pregnant person should consider.

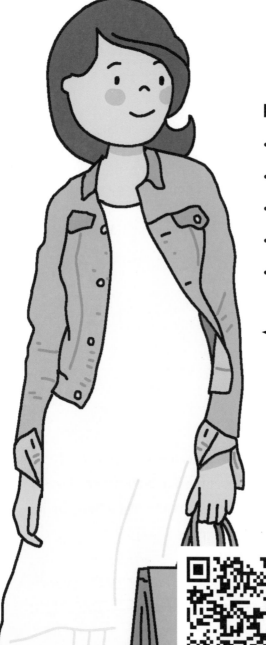

A loose-fitting jean jacket works with almost anything.

Comfy, casual dress, either loose or formfitting.

Mommy Hack

Consider pieces that can be used after delivery. Look for pieces with easy nursing access if you plan to breastfeed.

KEY POINTS

- Comfort is key.

- Look for pieces that will grow with you.

- Think soft, stretchy, and breathable.

- Choose clothes with elastic waistbands.

- Accessorize to spruce up your outfit.

GET THE RIGHT STUFF!

Scan the QR code to easily get our recommendations to find fashion basics that you will love.

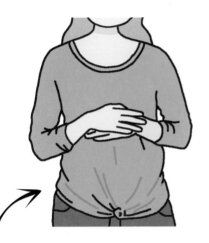

Loose and soft neutrals, long- and short-sleeve tees.

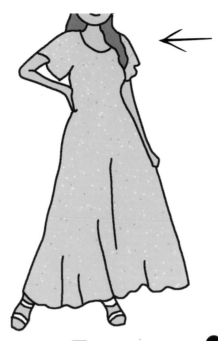

A maxi dress, loose and airy, if you want to hide your bump.

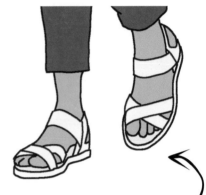

An absolute must is a pair of comfy slip-on flats or sandals.

the basics

10 FASHION PIECES THAT SHOULD BE IN BABY MAMA'S CLOSET

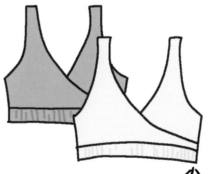

Super comfy nursing or sports bra.

An oversized sweater.

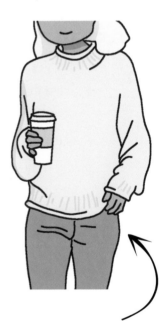

A pair of boyfriend/hubby jeans or maternity jeans

A pair of black yoga pants over the bump, paired with an oversized white button-down shirt.

MATERNITY CLOTHING
WHAT YOU WILL NEED

Want to buy some maternity clothes? Here are a few tips that you should know.

WHAT IS IT?

MATERNITY CLOTHING: Clothing made for pregnant women, which is designed to allow for changes in a woman's body as her pregnancy progresses.

DO YOU NEED THEM?

The answer is: it depends. Some woman can wear regular, oversized clothing, and it works for them, while others find it uncomfortable or find it hard to put together an outfit.

CLOTHING SIZING

Maternity clothing is sized the same as regular clothing sizes. For example, if you wear a size 8 in regular clothing, you will be a size 8 in maternity clothing.

Everyone's body is different, and so is every pregnancy; in addition, as with all clothing, sizing may vary by brand and retailer.

MATERNITY BRA SIZING

The general rule of thumb is:

Add one to two cup sizes and one back size to your pre-pregnancy size.

Don't be surprised if your shoe size goes up one size during pregnancy. Your ribs and hips may also become wider. Unfortunately, these changes may be permanent.

Fit and comfort are important, but how do you figure out what size to get in maternity clothes?

THE GENERAL RULE:

Whatever your size in regular clothing will be your size in maternity clothing.

EXAMPLE:

SIZE 8
IN REGULAR CLOTHING

=

SIZE 8
IN MATERNITY CLOTHING

GET THE RIGHT FIT

It is highly recommended that before buying a maternity bra you get fitted by an expert at your local lingerie store.

Check the maternity clothing size chart of a retailer to confirm the size.

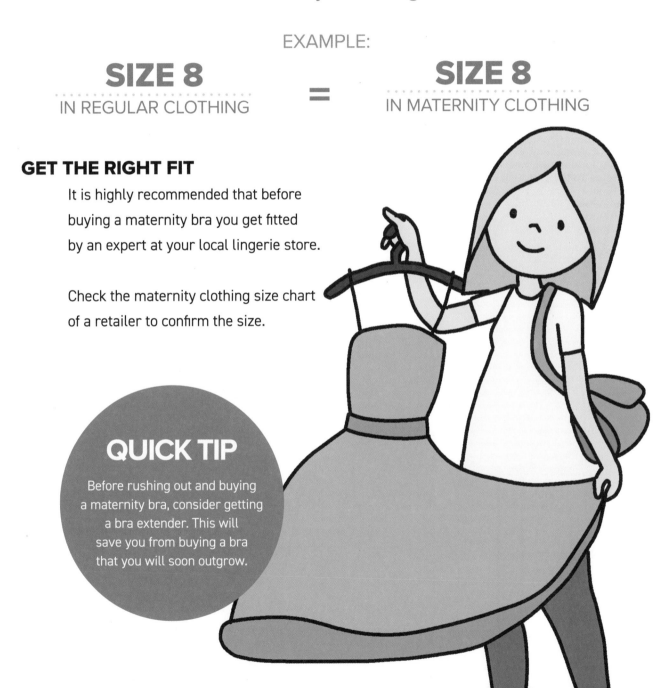

QUICK TIP

Before rushing out and buying a maternity bra, consider getting a bra extender. This will save you from buying a bra that you will soon outgrow.

SWELL!
PREGNANCY AND SWELLING

Your shoes and rings are starting to get a bit snug; swelling, while uncomfortable, is a common part of pregnancy.

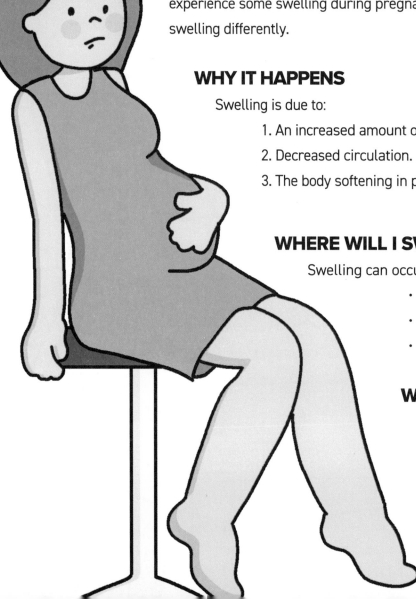

QUICK TIP
When approaching the second trimester, consider removing your rings before it is too late and you can't remove them.

OVERVIEW

In the second trimester, especially in the later part of the trimester, you may start noticing swelling, which typically will continue through the third trimester. It's normal to experience some swelling during pregnancy; however, everyone experiences swelling differently.

WHY IT HAPPENS

Swelling is due to:

1. An increased amount of blood and fluids in your body.
2. Decreased circulation.
3. The body softening in preparation for birth.

WHERE WILL I SWELL?

Swelling can occur anywhere, but generally occurs in the:

- Feet
- Legs
- Hands
- Vulva
- Ankles

WHEN TO BE CONCERNED?

If you experience any of the following symptoms, you should contact your doctor

- Headaches
- Blurry vision
- Pain in your upper right side

TIPS FOR REDUCING SWELLING

ELEVATE YOUR FEET

Elevating your legs when sitting will help your circulation.

DON'T STAND OR SIT FOR LONG PERIODS

Avoid long periods of standing or sitting. If you stand a lot, sit down once in a while; if you sit for long periods, get up and walk a bit.

COMPRESSION STOCKINGS

Wearing compression stockings or tights can help a bit with swelling.

STAY COOL

Staying out of the heat is recommended, as heat tends to make swelling worse.

COLD COMPRESSES

Apply cold compresses to vaginal swelling to ease some of your discomfort.

REDUCE EXTRA SALT

Cut down salt intake, as salt causes fluid retention and makes swelling worse.

MASSAGE

Gentle massage of swollen areas can help circulate the fluids that have accumulated.

SLEEP ON YOUR SIDE

Lying on your side, especially your left side, may ease swelling.

MOVE

Get appropriate pregnancy exercise, like walking or swimming, to help circulation.

DRINK PLENTY OF FLUIDS

Getting plenty of fluids and staying hydrated can help reduce swelling.

WEAR COMFORTABLE, LOOSE CLOTHING

Avoid tight clothing, especially around the wrists and ankles. Wear comfortable shoes and avoid high heels.

STRETCH MARKS
THE 411 ON THESE

The majority of women experience stretch marks, and although there is no magic formula to prevent them, there may be some things you can do to minimize them.

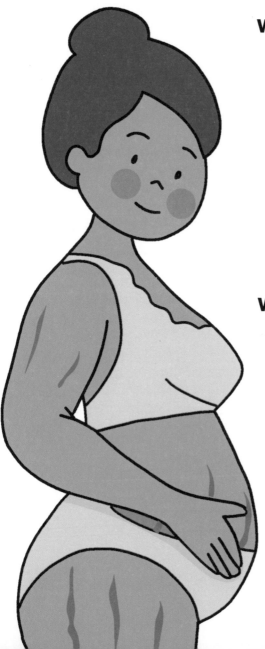

WHAT ARE THEY?

STRETCH MARKS: Narrow pink to purple lines that can develop on the skin's surface. They usually appear on the:

- Stomach
- Lower back
- Upper thighs
- Hips
- Butt
- Breasts

WHEN DOES IT HAPPEN?

These harmless lines are the result of overstretching the skin. Stretch marks usually appear in the third trimester as your baby bump expands.

After delivery, as your skin slowly shrinks, most stretch marks fade to white. Where you get stretch marks has a lot to do with the elasticity of your skin.

LOTIONS & OILS

Use lotions made with coconut oil, olive oil, beeswax, or vitamin E, or use shea or cocoa butter creams.

NUTRITION

Eating foods such as fruits and vegetables and taking your prenatal vitamins helps promote healthy skin.

HYDRATION

Keeping your skin well hydrated with water may help eliminate some of the stretching.

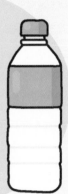

TIPS FOR MINIMIZING STRETCH MARKS

There is no proven way to prevent stretch marks, but you may be able to help minimize their appearance or development.

LASER THERAPY

After delivery you may consider laser therapy, where a laser penetrates the deep layers of skin stimulating collagen creation.

COLLAGEN

Taking collagen supplements may help minimize stretch marks.

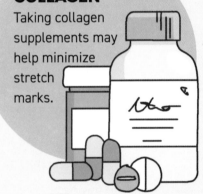

CONTROL THE CALORIES

Rapid weight gain can contribute to developing stretch marks.

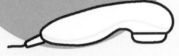

VITAMIN C

Getting enough vitamin C-rich food in your diet from oranges, strawberries, kale, bell peppers, and lemons may help.

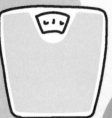

BELLY MASSAGE

Light belly massage might help improve your skin's elasticity.

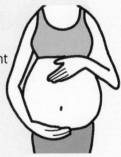

SOCK IT TO ME
COMPRESSION SOCKS, HOSE, AND MORE

Swelling can be common during pregnancy; compression socks or hosiery can help alleviate some of it.

WHAT IS IT?

COMPRESSION SOCKS OR HOSE: These are specially designed garments that apply gentle pressure to your legs and ankles to help prevent excess water becoming trapped in the body's tissue and to aid blood flow.

BENEFITS

- Improves blood circulation.
- Helps prevent blood clots.
- Reduces varicose veins.
- Lessens pain.
- Reduces swelling.
- Helps reduce spider veins.

WHEN TO WEAR?

You can start wearing compression socks or hose during any trimester, but during the second and third trimester you might need them more because swelling typically is greatest at this time.

DETERMINE COMPRESSION LEVEL

The compression should be comfortable—the fabric should not dig into your skin. Speak to your health-care provider to get their recommendation for what the correct level of compression is for you.

NOTE: Always speak to your health-care provider to understand the risks and benefits with using any treatment to determine that it is right for you and your baby.

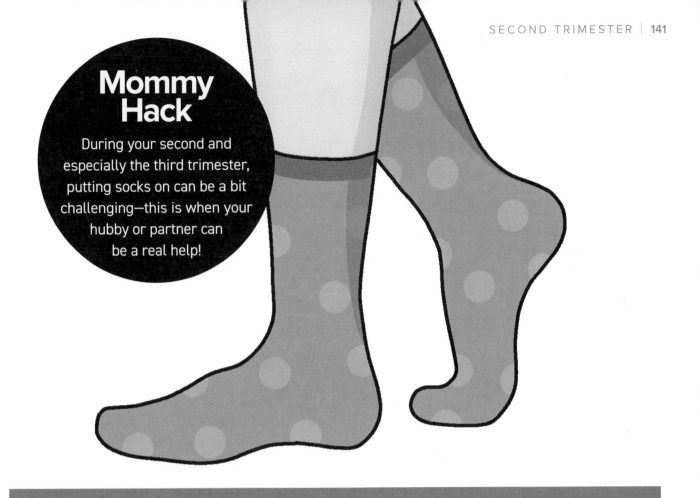

Mommy Hack

During your second and especially the third trimester, putting socks on can be a bit challenging—this is when your hubby or partner can be a real help!

COMPRESSION SOCKS | What to Know

Choose the size you would when picking a regular pair of socks or pantyhose.

LENGTHS:

BELOW THE KNEE
Reduces swelling of calves, ankles, and feet.

THIGH HIGH STOCKING
Improves circulation of the legs.

PANTYHOSE
Waist-high compression for legs and hips.

TYPES:

ANTI-EMBOLISM SOCKS
Maintains circulation and helps prevents blood clots.

GRADUATED SOCKS
Tighter around the ankles and looser toward the knees or thighs; improves circulation.

PRESSURES:

15-20 mmHg
Improves circulation without being too tight.

20-30 mmHg
Tighter; can help reduce varicose and spider veins.

30-40 mmHg
Can help with blood clots, severe swelling, and severe varicose veins.

EPSOM SALT BATHS
EASE THE ACHES AND PAINS

Being pregnant comes with a host of aches and pains, and an Epsom salt bath might help; but before adding Epsom salt to your bath, consult your doctor.

WHAT IS IT?

EPSOM SALT: Unlike regular salt, it is crystallized magnesium and sulfate. When placed in water, the crystals break down, and it is believed, when you soak in it, these components are absorbed through the skin.

EPSOM SALT BATH | HOW TO:

1 Fill the bath with lukewarm water, NOT HOT! water

2 Add two cups of Epsom salt to the bath, and allow it to dissolve.

3 Soak for around 15 minutes.

QUICK TIP

To avoid slipping and falling, make sure your tub has a nonslip mat in it and you have a nonslip mat on the floor. At this stage, your balance and center of gravity are likely to be a bit off.

WARNING

It is safe to take a bath while pregnant if you follow these four simple rules:

1. The water should never be too hot—it is dangerous for the baby.
2. Do not eat or drink the Epsom salt.
3. Do not add aromatic oils, like eucalyptus or lavender, to the bath.
4. Consult your doctor to make sure an Epsom salt bath is safe for you and your baby.

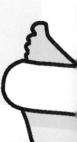

BENEFITS

SOOTHES ACHES & PAINS

Soaking in an Epsom salt bath can soothe sore muscles and back, hip, and joint pain.

REDUCES STRESS

Soaking in a warm Epsom salt bath may help relieve stress.

EASES HEMORRHOID PAIN

Developing hemorrhoids during pregnancy is very common, and soaking in an Epsom salt bath can help reduce hemorrhoid inflammation and discomfort.

REDUCES SWELLING

This can be great for swollen feet and ankles.

EASES CONSTIPATION

Soaking in an Epsom salt bath may help relieve constipation, which is very common during pregnancy.

REDUCES ITCHING

Epsom salts can help soothe skin and relieve itching.

EASES SEVERE MORNING SICKNESS

Adding Epsom salt to the bath has been known to help ease severe morning sickness for some.

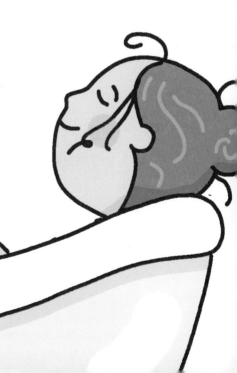

PREGNANCY PILLOWS

A GOOD NIGHT'S SLEEP

Choosing the right pregnancy pillow can be difficult; there are so many to choose from. Ultimately, it's a personal choice. Here are some things to help you decide.

QUICK TIP

When buying a pregnancy pillow, look for one that has a removable, machine-washable cover.

WHAT IS IT?

PREGNANCY PILLOW: These are specially designed pillows to support a pregnant person's body; they alleviate pain and help you get a better night's sleep. They provide very good support of the belly, back, and hips.

BENEFITS

1. ALLEVIATES ACHES & PAINS

As mom-to-be's body continues to grow in size and weight, it causes pain in the back, hips, shoulders, neck, and legs. A pregnancy pillow provides relief by helping to keep your spine in proper alignment.

2. IMPROVES CIRCULATION

It is recommended that pregnant moms sleep on their side to promote circulation. With your growing belly, this can be rather uncomfortable. A pregnancy pillow cushions and supports you, making sleeping on your side more comfortable.

3. BETTER NIGHT'S SLEEP

A pregnancy pillow eases your aching body, allowing you to get a better night's sleep.

4. HELPS WITH BREASTFEEDING

After delivery, the pregnancy pillow can be used to support your baby during breastfeeding.

Mommy Hack

Some moms found the pregnancy pillow also worked well as a nursing pillow.

TOP PREGNANCY PILLOWS

BENEFITS

C-SHAPED

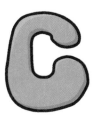
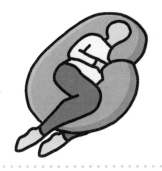

- Supports your back and belly.
- Keep legs and hips aligned.
- Supports the neck.
- Supports proper spine alignment.

U-SHAPED

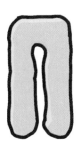
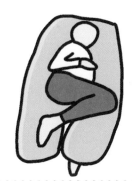

- Supports the whole body.
- Keeps legs and hips aligned.
- Supports the neck.
- Supports proper spine alignment.

J-SHAPED

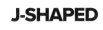
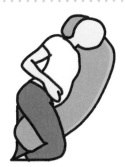

- Supports the belly.
- Keeps legs and hips aligned.
- Supports the neck.

WEDGE

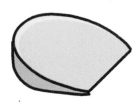
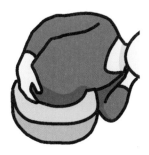

- Supports areas of your choosing.
- Prevents rolling over in sleep.
- Is cooler than other pillows.

EXTRA NOTE

SLEEPING HOT: If you generally sleep hot, consider avoiding synthetic covers.

SUPPORT: Polyfill pillows are softer and more adjustable. Memory foam-filled pillows provide firmer support.

LYING ON YOUR BACK

WHAT'S OK, AND WHAT'S NOT?

As if getting comfortable was not hard enough, you also need to be aware that lying on your back can potentially cause problems—here is why.

OVERVIEW

As your belly grows (during the second and third trimesters), lying flat on your back becomes a concern because it puts weight and pressure on your spine and the major blood vessel (inferior vena cava) that carries blood to your uterus. The longer you lie on your back, the greater the possibility of this happening.

WHAT TO DO

The American College of Obstetricians and Gynecologists recommends:

- Sleeping on your side during the second and third trimesters.
- Bending one or both knees.
- Placing a pillow between your knees and another under your belly.

ADDITIONAL ADVICE

- Place a pillow on the mattress behind your back; this will help prevent rolling onto your back.
- After week 20, do not spend extended periods lying on your back.
- Don't lie flat—try to lie at a 30-to-40 degree angle.

QUICK TIP

It is recommended that you try and sleep on your left side to take pressure off the inferior vena cava (a major vein in the body), which is on the right side.

Mommy Hack

MAKE THE SWITCH

You can make your life just a little bit easier if you take the side of the bed that is closer to the bathroom, for nighttime peeing.

NOTE: The information provided is not a substitute for professional medical advice, diagnosis, or treatment. Always consult your obstetrician or primary health-care provider to ensure that a treatment or medication is right and safe for you and your baby.

2ND TRIMESTER CONCERNS

WHAT YOU NEED TO KNOW

Even though this period is one which typically has few aches and pains, there are some complications to watch for.

OVERVIEW

The second trimester is the period when most people feel most comfortable; nausea and vomiting have eased, and the risk of miscarriage is reduced.

CONCERNS TO SHARE WITH YOUR DOCTOR

VAGINAL BLEEDING

While miscarriage is less common at this time, it still can happen. In some cases, bleeding can be a symptom of a miscarriage.

PRETERM LABOR

Experiencing labor pain before the 37th week is known as preterm labor. Preterm labor can be triggered by:

- A bladder infection
- Diabetes
- Kidney disease
- Smoking
- History of preterm labor
- Twin pregnancy complications

CERVICAL INSUFFICIENCY

When the cervix (the tissue that connects the vagina to the uterus) opens and shortens in the second trimester. This can lead to preterm birth or pregnancy loss.

PPROM

In 2 to 3 percent of pregnancies, water breaks preterm (before 37 weeks). This is called preterm prelabor rupture of membranes (PPROM) and can lead to infection and preterm delivery.

PREECLASMPSIA

Preeclampsia is a serious blood pressure disorder that can happen during pregnancy or postpartum. Symptoms can include persistent headache, seeing spots, blurry vision, swelling, shortness of breath, and abdominal pain.

INJURY

Pregnant people are more prone to losing their balance, as their center of gravity has literally shifted. Care should be taken around slippery areas, like bathrooms.

BREATHING ISSUES

You might find yourself short of breath due to pressure placed on your lungs by your growing baby. You may also notice that you are experiencing a stuffy nose, nosebleeds, and snoring. This is caused by increased blood flow to the lining of your nose, which causes swelling.

GESTATIONAL DIABETES

As your baby grows, so does baby's demand for more nutrition, which can raise your glucose levels and increase the risk of a difficult pregnancy.

BLEEDING GUMS

Bleeding gums is a common problem due to hormonal changes in the body. Pregnant persons with dental issues are more likely to deliver a low-birth-weight baby or go into preterm labor.

HEMORRHOIDS

Varicose veins in the anus that become enlarged due to increased blood flow. They itch and can be painful.

You're rocking
that baby bump.

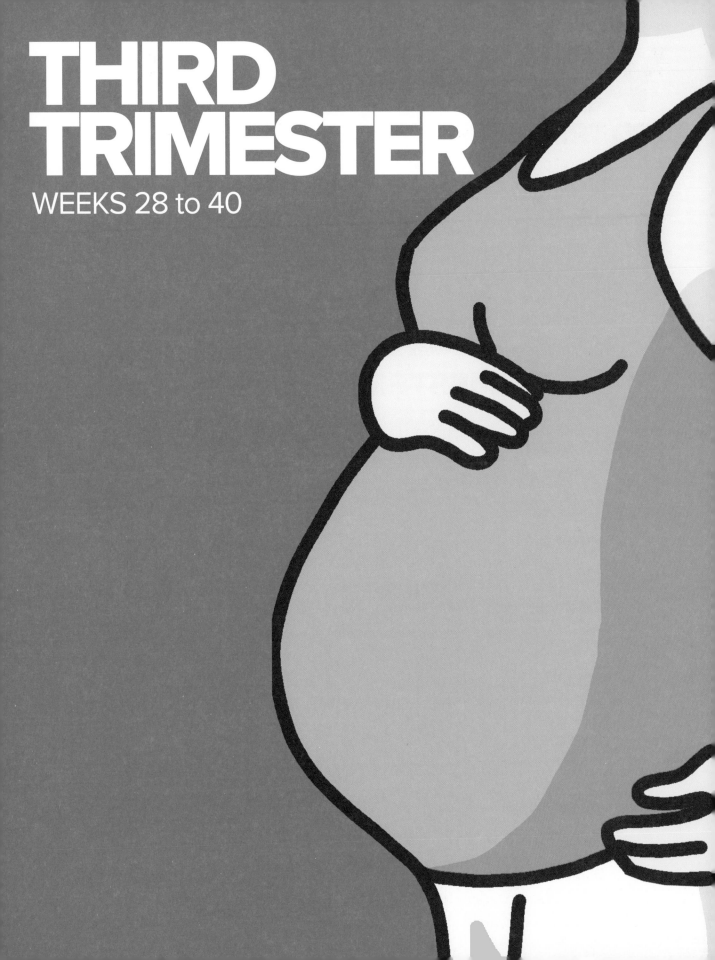

THIRD TRIMESTER

WEEKS 28 to 40

YOUR BODY
3RD TRIMESTER: WEEKS 28 to 40

The last phase of pregnancy; you are on the home stretch now.

OVERVIEW

Your baby will continue to grow and develop to full maturity during this time. You are likely to feel more uncomfortable as baby and you continue to grow.

HOW LONG WILL IT LAST?

This phase begins at week 28 and lasts until birth or three months.

3rd TRIMESTER (WEEKS 28 to 40)

WHAT'S NEW?

BABY BUMP:

Your baby bump just keeps getting bigger.

MOVEMENT:

You should feel lots of activity from your baby at this point.

BRAXTON-HICKS CONTRACTIONS:

You may have false labor contractions as your body begins preparing for delivery.

EMOTIONS:

You may feel more emotional as you near your labor/delivery date.

SWELLING:

The swelling you started to experience in the second trimester continues.

HEMORRHOIDS:

Varicose veins of the anus may develop or continue from the second trimester.

BREASTS:

Breasts continue to grow, and you may experience some leakage.

TINGLING & NUMBNESS:

The swelling in your body may press on nerves, causing tingling and numbness in the legs, arms, and hands. The skin on your belly may feel numb from being stretched so much.

VARICOSE VEINS:

You may develop bluish, swollen veins beneath the skin of the calves or inside of the thighs.

PAIN IN THE BACK, PELVIS, & HIPS:

As your baby continues to grow, the stress on your back also grows. You may experience pain in your hips and pelvis as the joints relax in preparation for delivery.

SHORTNESS OF BREATH:

The pressure on your lungs will continue as your baby grows, potentially causing difficulty breathing.

WEIGHT GAIN:

You will continue to add weight, which will slow and even out as you near delivery.

HAIR:

The hair on your arms, legs, and face may begin to grow due to hormonal stimulation.

VAGINAL DISCHARGE:

White-colored discharge (leukorrhea) might increase and contain more mucus.

STRETCH MARKS:

As baby grows, your skin will continue to stretch and may result in stretch marks on the stomach, breasts, thighs, or butt.

BODY TEMPERATURE:

As baby grows and radiates heat, you might feel increasingly hot.

SKIN:

Dry, itchy skin, particularly on the stomach, may continue. Dark patches may develop on your face.

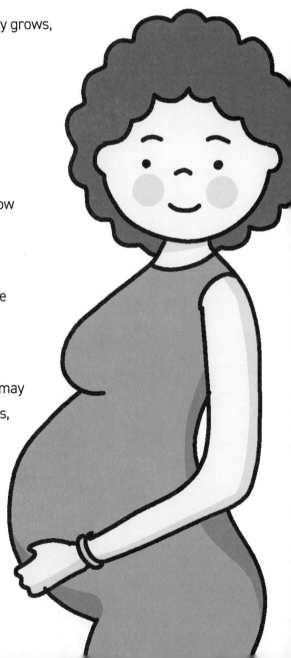

YOUR BABY
THE 3RD TRIMESTER

OVERVIEW

Your baby continues to grow in size and weight:

- Adding two to three more pounds to reach a total weight of between six and nine pounds.
- Growing in length to between 18 and 20 inches.

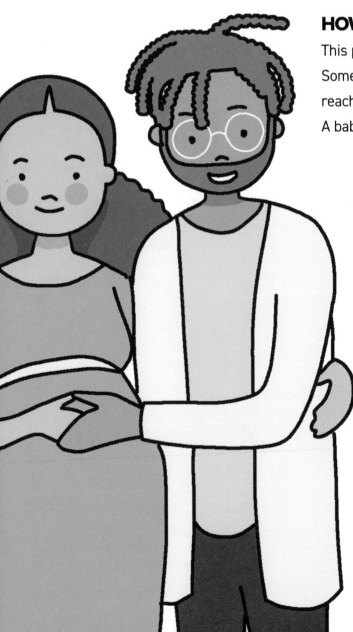

HOW LONG WILL IT LAST?

This phase begins week 28 and continues to week 40. Some pregnancies go past the 40-week mark, but if you reach week 41 or 42, you are considered overdue. A baby is considered full-term at 39 weeks.

WHAT'S NEW?

SENSES:

The baby's senses are in their final stage of development. Earlier your baby's eyes were fused shut; now they can open and sense light. Baby's hearing is beginning to develop.

BRAIN:

The baby's brain continues to develop and mature.

WEIGHT:

Your baby will gain about one-half pound every week.

BONES:

Baby's bones are hardening, except for its skull bones, which remain soft for the delivery.

POSITIONING:

The baby will begin to turn head down in preparation for delivery.

WEEK	SIZE	WHAT IS HAPPENING
WK. 28	14.8 in. Eggplant	Baby is able to open and close its eyes and sense light. Eyelashes have formed.
WK. 29	15.2 in. Acorn Squash	Muscles continue to develop, and the head grows to make room for the developing brain.
WK. 30	15.7 in. Cabbage	Baby may be kicking a lot now, as your womb is getting increasingly tighter as baby grows.
WK. 31	16.2 in. Coconut	Baby will be getting input from all five senses. Baby can begin to regulate its body temperature.
WK. 32	16.7 in. Pineapple	Baby's transparent skin is becoming opaque.
WK. 33	17.2 in. Durian Fruit	A coating called vernix caseosa is forming to protect baby's skin.
WK. 34	17.7 in. Butternut Squash	Baby likely will start turning into a head down position.
WK. 35	18.2 in. Swiss Chard	Lungs are almost fully developed.
WK. 36	18.7 in. Honeydew	Baby will begin to shed the vernix (the waxy substance that protects its skin).
WK. 37	19.1 in. Winter Melon	The lanugo (tiny soft hairs that cover the baby) is almost gone.
WK. 38	19.6 in. Pumpkin	Meconium (baby's first poop) begins to build up in baby's intestines.
WK. 39	20 in. Jackfruit	If baby is born now, it is considered full-term.
WK. 40	20.2 in. Watermelon	If you are still pregnant, don't worry; it is not uncommon to go past one's delivery date.

THE MUST-HAVES

THIRD TRIMESTER

Practical suggestions for common pregnancy issues.

Mommy Hack

Buy maternity clothing secondhand and pass them on when you are done with them; it's a great way to save money.

GET THE RIGHT STUFF!

Scan the QR code to easily get our recommendations for the essentials you may need for the third trimester.

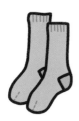

COMPRESSION SOCKS or HOSE

Make sure they provide a tight but comfortable fit. There are several styles, but the most effective are knee-highs or pantyhose. They come in different levels of compression depending on the amount of swelling. Speak to your doctor about the right level of compression for you.

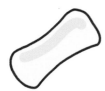

PANTY LINERS

You may experience increased vaginal discharge and, with all that pressure on your bladder as baby grows, you may have leakage, making a panty liner a good idea. Consider reusable panty liners if you want to save money and avoid waste.

NURSING PADS

You can start leaking in your third trimester, and 8 to 12 nursing pads that are soft, absorbent, and made of organic cotton can be handy. Pads come in three types: disposables, reusable cotton, or silicone pads.

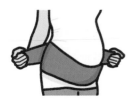

MATERNITY BELTS & SUPPORTS

Depending on how severe your hip and back pain is, you might need a little extra support, and a maternity belt might do the trick. These devices wrap around your body, from your lower back to your belly, offering better weight and posture support. There are many different styles.

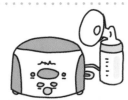

BREAST PUMP or PUMPING BRA

If you plan on breastfeeding, you will want to get your pump ahead of time.

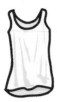

OVERSIZED SWEATERS OR SHIRTS

These loose-fitting tops are essential. They are super comfy—you may even find yourself wearing them after you give birth.

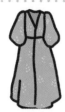

LOOSE DRESSES

Having a maxi dress that is soft and stretchy is perfect; you'll look good but still be super comfy. Having a few maternity dresses is also nice. They should be lightweight, flexible, and breathable with no complicated fasteners.

MORE HEALTH SNACKS

You are going to be hungry; having healthy snacks handy is a must. Try high-protein snacks or bars.

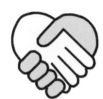

CHIROPRACTIC/PRENATAL P.T. CARE

For severe pain, consider seeing a chiropractor or prenatal physical therapist for an adjustment or prenatal massage. Be sure to get the approval of your doctor, and tell the chiropractor or massage therapist that you are pregnant.

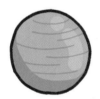

BIRTHING BALL

Birthing balls are made of extra-thick material. Make sure that yours is made of a durable material and that it is the right size for you.

BINDER OF DOCUMENTS

Have all your documents organized in a binder so that when you go to the hospital you have all the required documents for admittance and delivery.

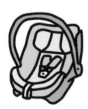

CAR SEAT

Look for models that have a five-point harness (two shoulder straps, two waist straps, and one strap between the legs) and padding around the head for side-impact protection. Ideally, it should be able to grow with your child and be compatible with the current car LATCH system.

THANK-YOU NOTES

If you are having a shower, you will want to have either thank-you cards that you can mail or be prepared to send them digitally.

CHILDBIRTH CLASSES

GETTING STARTED

One of the most helpful things you and your partner can do while pregnant is attend childbirth classes.

QUICK TIP

Be sure to check your insurance, as it may cover some or all of the expense of classes. Without insurance, classes range from **$50 to $200.**

WHAT IS IT?

BIRTHING CLASSES: These classes help prepare you and your partner for childbirth. They offer information about what you can expect during pregnancy, labor, delivery, and the postpartum period. Some classes are primarily lectures, while in others you participate and receive more one-on-one coaching.

WHEN TO ATTEND?

Most parents-to-be begin childbirth classes in the third trimester, around month seven.

TYPES OF CLASSES

There are several different types of childbirth classes, each with a specific focus and philosophy. Many of these classes can be attended in person or have online options available.

The major types of classes are:

1. Lamaze
2. Bradley Method
3. Alexander Technique
4. HypnoBirthing

HOW TO FIND THE RIGHT CLASS FOR YOU

- Your doctor, midwife, nurse, or doula
- Friends and family
- Hospitals, pregnancy centers, birth centers
- Your local community resource center
- Online searches

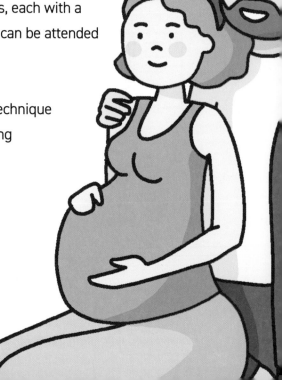

MAJOR TYPES OF CLASSES

Although these are the well-known types of classes, there are many other options focused on a variety of needs; for example, there are classes for fathers, classes for LGBTQ families, etc.

LAMAZE:

The most widely used childbirth classes, Lamaze teaches natural childbirth coping methods, utilizing instruction on specific comforting, relaxation, and breathing techniques.

Lamaze does not support or discourage the use of medicines or medical interventions during labor and delivery but focuses on providing the options available, letting the mom-to-be make the decision that is best for her. They also teach baby care and breastfeeding.

BRADLEY METHOD:

This method emphasizes birth as a natural process; it encourages moms-to-be to trust their bodies and focus on diet and exercise. It prepares moms-to-be for delivery without pain medications and prepares partners to be a labor coach.

ALEXANDER TECHNIQUE:

This method focuses on releasing muscular tension, improved breathing, coordination, and calming oneself utilizing improved body posture and movement.

HYPNOBIRTHING/HYPNOBABY:

This method utilizes a mixture of medical-grade self-hypnosis, relaxation, visualization, meditation, and breathing techniques to manage pain. You will also learn about baby-care techniques and breastfeeding.

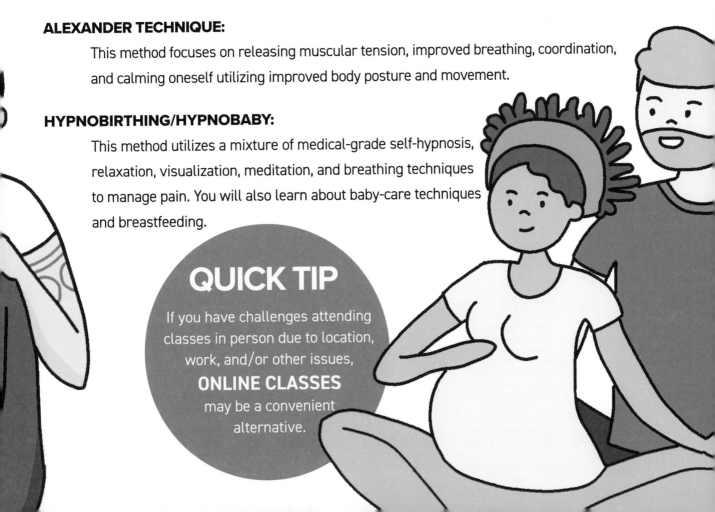

QUICK TIP

If you have challenges attending classes in person due to location, work, and/or other issues, **ONLINE CLASSES** may be a convenient alternative.

IT'S A WRAP
GETTING A LITTLE SUPPORT

We all need a little support now and then, including your third trimester; we'll have a look at some handy devices that might just do the trick.

QUICK TIP

As your belly grows, it's not uncommon to experience some numbness or tingling of the abdominal skin.

WHAT ARE THEY, AND WHAT'S THE DIFFERENCE?

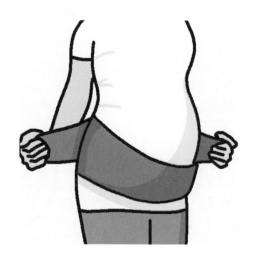

BELLY BELT:

A rigid, adjustable belt that wraps around the belly. They provide added support for the lower back, pelvis, hips, and abdomen. They are usually worn over clothing.

EXTENDED WEAR:

Wearing a belly belt for long periods of time might weaken muscles, as you may become too dependent on the device. Check the manufacturer's recommended amount of time for wearing it, and speak to your doctor about the amount of time that's right for you.

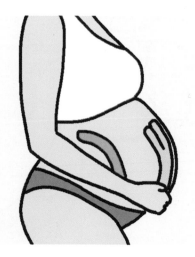

KINESIOLOGY TAPE:

Kinesiology tape or spider tape can provide posture support and ease aches and pains associated with a growing belly. These products provide support and can be worn under clothing.

PRENATAL OR MATERNITY CRADLE:

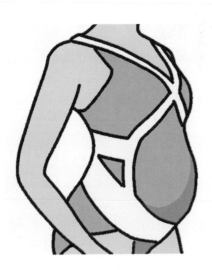

These consist of a belly belt that wraps around the lower body with an upper strap that extends around and over the belly, essentially cradling the belly.

Many of these come as separate pieces, so you can wear only the belly belt or add the additional strap if you need more support.

MATERNITY UNDERWEAR:

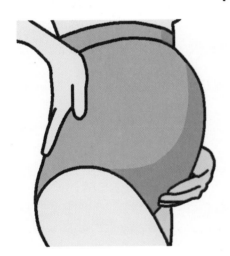

These undergarments are designed with an underbelly supportive belt and nonbinding waistbands to support the pelvis and hips. They provide enough stretch to grow with your growing bump and support the pelvis and hips.

There are several versions:

- Above-the-bump
- Below-the-bump
- Mid-bump

MATERNITY LEGGINGS:

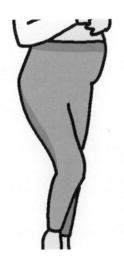

These leggings are designed to provide added underbelly support; they have just enough stretch to allow for your growing bump. They come in several versions:

- Above-the-bump
- Low-rise fits (under the bump)
- Foldable bands (can go over or under the bump)

HOSPITAL BAG

IT'S IN THE BAG

Having a baby is stressful enough, so having your bag packed and ready to go before you are rushing out the door avoids having to run around at the last minute trying to pull it all together.

WHAT IS IT?

HOSPITAL BAG: The bag you will take to the hospital when you go to deliver your baby. It contains all the various things you will need during your labor, delivery, and recovery.

WHEN TO PACK?

Don't wait till the last minute; have your bag packed and ready to go between weeks 32 and 35.

Mommy Hack

Having an extra-long power cord to charge your phone with can be very, very helpful; you may have a difficult time reaching with a shorter/regular one.

HOSPITAL BAG
PACKED & READY TO GO
WEEKS **32–35**

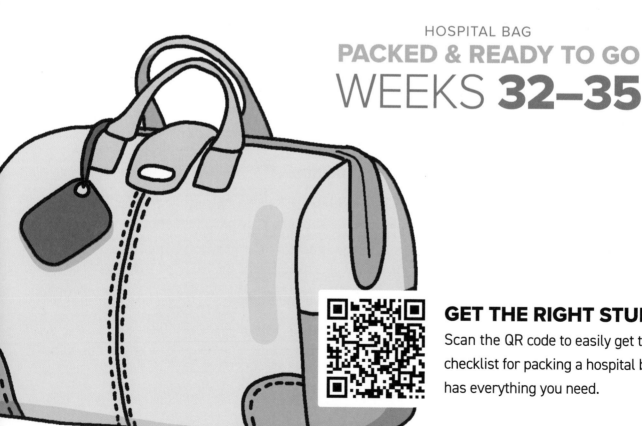

GET THE RIGHT STUFF!

Scan the QR code to easily get the best checklist for packing a hospital bag that has everything you need.

HOSExPITAL BAG LABOR CHECKLIST

 DOCUMENTS: Your ID, insurance information, and birth plan (a few copies).

 BATHROBE: A super comfortable robe.

 SOCKS: A couple of pairs of comfy nonskid socks.

 SLIPPERS & FLIP-FLOPS: To wear in the shower.

 LIP BALM: Your lips will become dry during delivery.

 LOTION: Some body lotion or massage oil for a massage to ease sore muscles.

 SPRAY BOTTLE: You may get hot during delivery, and a nice spritz might help cool you off.

 PILLOW, SHEET, & BLANKET: Having your own more comfortable pillow and blanket can be comforting.

 ENTERTAINMENT: Your favorite music or other entertainment to distract you and pass the time.

 EYE MASK: For labor and after delivery.

 HAIR TIES: Have some hair ties or headbands.

 TOILETRIES: Toothbrush, travel-size toothpaste, mouthwash, deodorant, shampoo, and conditioner.

 HAIRBRUSH: Your hairbrush and/or comb.

 EYE CARE: Bring your glasses, contacts, lens case, and contact solution.

 MEDICATIONS: Be sure to bring any prescription medications.

 WATER BOTTLE: Take a reusable water bottle.

 HARD CANDY: Sugar-free hard candy to alleviate dry mouth and freshen your breath.

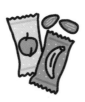 **SNACKS:** Something to nibble on if approved by your doctor.

HOSPITAL BAG
IT'S IN THE BAG

HOSPITAL BAG POST-DELIVERY **CHECKLIST**

 NIGHTGOWN: A comfy, loose gown, one that is easy to open in front for breastfeeding.

 MATERNITY PADS: Heavy flow, thick and long sanitary pads, or adult diapers.

 UNDERWEAR: Several pairs of postpartum underwear.

 NURSING BRAS/TANKS: Support for swollen, tender breasts.

 PHONE CHARGER: Make sure you have chargers for your phone, laptop, and/or tablet.

 CLOTHING: If you want to lose the gown, try some maternity yoga pants and tops. Keep them loose and comfortable.

 MORE SNACKS: Nutritious nibbles like crackers, granola, apple, nuts, etc. if you get the munchies.

 NIPPLE CREAM: In case your nipples get chapped.

 TOWEL: Hospital towels are not the softest; consider bringing your own bath towel and washcloth.

 PERINEAL SPRAY: Your call; the hospital may give you one or you can bring your own.

 TOILETRIES: Toothbrush, travel-size toothpaste, mouthwash, deodorant, shampoo, and conditioner.

 NURSING PADS: To absorb any leaks.

 WET WIPES: Having these for little cleanups can be handy.

 COSMETICS: Some makeup or whatever might make you feel good.

HOSPITAL BAG PARTNER CHECKLIST

SNACKS: Having some yummy treats is nice to keep your energy up. Have some change for vending machines.

PHONE & CAMERA: Have your phone or camera ready.

CHARGERS: Make sure you have chargers for your phone, laptop, and/or tablet.

CLOTHING: You may want a change of clothes and something to sleep in.

ENTERTAINMENT: Soothing music, games, books, magazines, whatever you'll need.

MEDICATION: Medication that you normally take.

CORD BANKING KIT: Be sure to bring it with you, if banking tissue or cord blood.

TOILETRIES: Toothbrush, travel-size toothpaste, tissues, mouthwash, deodorant, shampoo, and conditioner.

PILLOW & BLANKET: Having your own more comfortable pillow and blanket can be nice.

HOSPITAL BAG BABY CHECKLIST

CAR SEAT: A must-have; you can't leave the hospital without one.

BABY OUTFIT: Weather-appropriate clothing, with socks or booties to take the baby home in.

PEDIATRICIAN INFO: Just in case it is needed.

BABY BLANKET: The hospital may give you one, but it's best to be prepared.

BABY HAT: Babies lose a lot of heat from their heads, so cover it to keep them warm.

BABY SHOWER
TIME TO CELEBRATE!

Definitely one of the fun aspects of having a baby.

GET YOUR <u>FREE</u> SHOWER PLANNER

Scan the QR code to get our baby shower planner and list of everything you need to organize the perfect baby shower.

WHAT IS IT?

A BABY SHOWER: A party thrown to celebrate the birth of a new baby. It's an opportunity for friends and family to express their joy and give gifts and the things baby will need to mom-to-be.

WHEN SHOULD IT BE DONE?

There is no right or wrong time to have a shower. Some prefer to have it before the baby is born, and others prefer to wait.

MOST BABY SHOWERS OCCUR
4–6 WEEKS
BEFORE THE BABY IS BORN

THROWING A SHOWER

- Select a date and time.
- Determine a guest list and budget.
- Choose a venue.
- Send invitations from the host.
- Plan a menu and decor.
- Determine what will happen at the party and when.

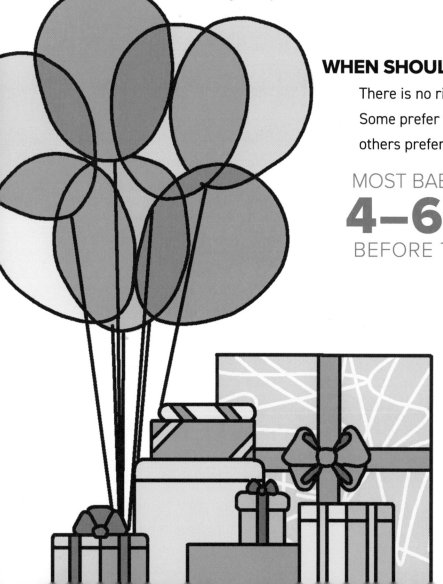
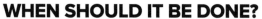

WHO DOES IT?

Typically, the baby shower is planned by friends or family, but it can be done by mom-to-be.

BABY REGISTRY

A baby registry or gift registry is typically created by the parents-to-be. It's a list of the things the expecting parents need. This helps gift-givers buy things that the parents-to-be want.

WHO ATTENDS?

Showers used to be an all-female event; today they have become increasingly a party for all members of the family and friends (male and female). The party can be quite large, or it can be small and intimate.

WHAT IS IT LIKE?

A baby shower can range from a fun and playful event to an elegant affair—it just depends on what the mom-to-be would like.

WHO PAYS FOR IT?

Typically, the host pays for the baby shower, but there is no right way to pay it. The cost can be shared by the family and friends who are hosting the party, or it can be the parents-to-be who pay for the event.

OPENING GIFTS

There is no right way to open presents, but they are typically opened during the event. Much of the fun comes from seeing the various gifts and clever wrappings. Gifts are usually opened toward the end of the party.

OTHER THINGS TO CONSIDER

FOOD: Baby showers can be as simple as a cake, or hors d'oeuvres, or a meal.
ACTIVITIES: At some showers, games are played and prizes given, but it's not a requirement.

BIRTH PLAN
TELL ME WHAT YOU WANT

The delivery and birth of your baby is a very special moment. To help ensure you get the delivery and birth you want, you need a birth plan.

GET YOUR <u>FREE</u> BIRTH PLANNER

Scan the QR code to get the ultimate birth plan so everybody knows what you want for your labor and delivery.

WHAT IS IT?

BIRTH PLAN: A written outline that tells your health-care team what you would like to happen before, during, and after labor and delivery.

It is very specific to **YOU**, your wants, your needs, your medical history, and the services available to you.

YOU DON'T ALWAYS GET WHAT YOU WANT

Depending on how your delivery progresses, it might impact your preferences. For example, if you want a vaginal delivery but you begin to experience complications, you might be required to have an emergency C-section. So, flexibility is important.

REVIEWING THE PLAN

Share your birth plan with your partner, doula, and doctor ahead of time to make sure all your preferences are possible and there are not any unforeseen complications.

WHAT TO PUT IN A BIRTH PLAN

- Your name and contact information.
- Your doctor's, midwife's, other health-care providers' names, and contact information.
- Who is your birth partner, if any, and what is their contact information?
- Who is your primary support person, and what is their contact information?

- Where you plan on giving birth.

- Whether you want anyone else in the delivery room, if possible, and who that is.

- Whether you want the lights dimmed, music playing.

- What position you'd like to be in during labor.

- If you want fetal monitoring done electronically or by stethoscope or fetoscope.

- Where you want to labor: a tub, shower, or a special facility like a birthing pool.

- If you have any particular feelings about using forceps or a vacuum.

- Whether there is anything in particular that will help you feel more relaxed.

- Whether you care how many people are in the room during labor.

- Are you interested in special facilities, like a birthing pool?

- Any particular feelings about a Vitamin K shot and eye drops.

- If you want the baby to sleep in your room or the nursery.

- If you want to wear your clothing or a hospital gown.

- Can staff use intermittent monitoring as long as it's safe?

- The type of pain management you want.

- If you would like to do skin-to-skin right after birth.

- If you are having a boy, do you want him circumcised?

- If you want a medicated or unmedicated delivery.

- Whether you would like to feed the baby after birth.

- Whether or not you want an episiotomy.

- Whether you want delayed cord clamping.

- If you want delayed bathing for the baby.

- If you want a mirror to watch the delivery.

- Who is going to cut the umbilical cord?

- If you want pictures or video taken.

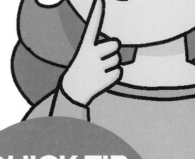

QUICK TIP

Make sure to share and review your birth plan with your doctor and delivery team up front, because once the delivery starts, the hospital staff tends to go on autopilot.

HEMORRHOIDS
WHAT A PAIN IN THE ASS

A common occurrence during pregnancy, nearly 50 percent of women will develop hemorrhoids.

WHAT IS IT?

HEMORRHOIDS: Swollen veins inside or outside the anus. They can be as small as a bead or as big as a grape.

Types of hemorrhoids:

INTERNAL: Hemorrhoids that form inside the rectum—these are usually painless but can cause bleeding. If an internal hemorrhoid extends outside of the rectum, that is called a "prolapse" and can cause pain.

EXTERNAL: Hemorrhoids that form outside of the rectum, near the anus. These can be highly sensitive and cause pain.

WHY DO THEY HAPPEN?

They are a result of:

- Increased blood flow in the pelvic area.
- Pressure from the growing baby.
- Hormonal changes.
- Constipation.

SYMPTOMS

- Bleeding
- A bump/raised skin area
- Swelling
- Pain when pooping
- Itching around the anus

Seeing any blood in your stool, or on toilet paper after having a bowel movement, can be scary, but bleeding from a hemorrhoid is usually harmless. Even so, it's always wise to let your health-care provider know about any bleeding.

WILL THEY GO AWAY?

Developing hemorrhoids during pregnancy is common, and they tend to go away after baby is born.

TREATMENT

You will want to treat your hemorrhoids to prevent them from getting worse. Here are some things you can do to help ease the pain.

WITCH HAZEL

Use wipes or pads with witch hazel.

EPSOM SALT BATH

Soaking in a warm Epsom salt bath for 10 minutes a couple times a day may help bring some relief.

GENTLE, GENTLE, GENTLE

Be gentle when cleaning/wiping yourself. You may choose to use wet, flushable wipes that are gentler on your skin.

SITZ BATH

Soaking in two to three inches of clean, warm water for 10 to 15 minutes at a time, a couple times a day, can soothe sore, swollen hemorrhoids.

LOOSEN UP THE POO

Drinking 8 to 12 8-ounce glasses of water a day, taking a stool softener, and eating a high-fiber diet can help ease constipation and keep stool soft.

TAKE THE PRESSURE OFF

Try not to stand or sit for extended periods of time; sit on a donut-shaped pillow and try not to strain when going number two.

EXERCISE

Doing Kegel exercises and getting regular, daily, pregnancy-appropriate exercise can help improve blood flow in your rectum.

MANAGE YOUR WEIGHT

Try not to gain more weight than recommended by your doctor.

NOTE: Always speak to your health-care provider about any treatment to understand the risks and benefits so that you and your baby are kept safe.

PAIN RELIEF
PAIN-MANAGEMENT PLAN/NON-MEDICATED

Everyone's experience of labor and delivery is different, but let's be real, you are delivering something the size of a watermelon, so you will have some pain. How each person handles that pain is hard to know. But it's important to have a plan in place before you deliver your baby.

WHAT IS IT?

NON-MEDICATED PAIN-MANAGEMENT PLAN: A plan to use medication-free techniques to manage or ease the pain of labor and delivery.

NON-MEDICATED OPTIONS

BREATHING TECHNIQUES

This method focuses on increased awareness of breathing and your body. It also strives to induce relaxation using meditation to help you keep calm. These techniques also help increase the flow of oxygen to the baby.

MOVEMENT AND POSITION CHANGES

By changing your position, you may experience less pain—for example, by sitting upright, standing, kneeling, or walking.

BIRTHING BALL

Also called a labor ball, it is an inflated rubber ball (similar to an exercise ball but slightly larger) that moms lean against or sit on to keep upright and active, which helps relieve the pain of labor. It also speeds labor and promotes baby's descent into the pelvis.

FOCUS/DISTRACTION

This technique relies on diverting your attention by focusing on other things. Distraction is essentially diverting your focus to various things around you: people, images, TV, etc. This method can be enhanced by verbal coaching, visualization, or self-hypnosis.

MUSIC

Music can help create a calm and soothing environment.

APPLYING HEAT OR COLD

Some laboring women experience pain relief from the application of heat or cold to different parts of the body, either separately or at the same time. Heat can be applied using a hot water bottle, hot moist towel, or warm blanket. Cold can be applied using an ice bag, washcloth soaked in ice water, or even a bag of frozen peas.

COUNTERPRESSURE

This technique helps alleviate back pain during labor. It is done by applying steady, strong pressure to painful spots on the lower back. It can also be done by applying pressure to the sides of the hips.

MASSAGE

Massaging various parts of the body by using light to firm stroking, vibration, kneading, circular pressure, or steady pressure can help ease labor pains.

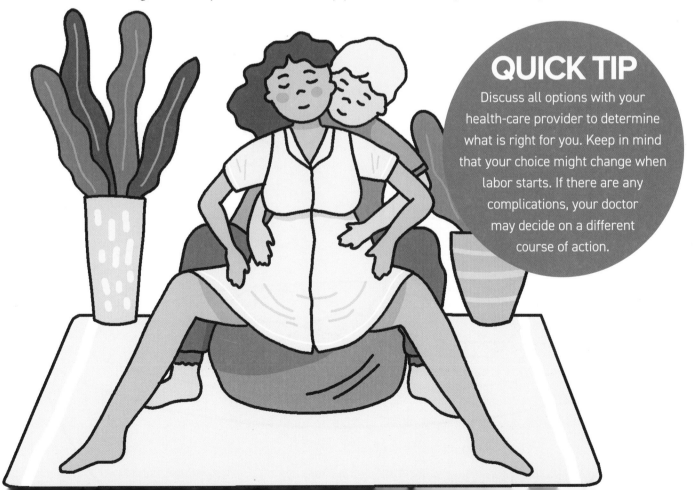

QUICK TIP

Discuss all options with your health-care provider to determine what is right for you. Keep in mind that your choice might change when labor starts. If there are any complications, your doctor may decide on a different course of action.

PAIN RELIEF
PAIN-MANAGEMENT PLAN/NON-MEDICATED

As we said in the first part of our discussion of non-medicated pain relief, everyone's experience of labor and delivery is different, but in addition to the techniques we just described, here are some more for you to consider.

NON-MEDICATED OPTIONS CONTINUED

HYDROTHERAPY

This technique uses immersion in warm water during labor to help soothe and relieve pain. The types of hydrotherapy range from sitting or floating in a warm bath (this is not a water birth; actual delivery does not take place in the tub).

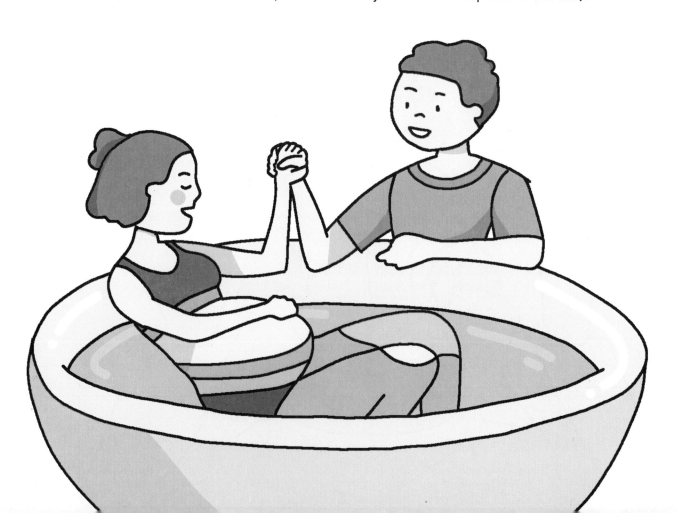

WARM SHOWER

Stand or sit in a shower, using a handheld massage shower head to spray yourself with warm water.

ACUPUNCTURE

This technique involves inserting super-thin needles through the skin at specific points on the body to reduce pain.

AROMATHERAPY

The use of essential oils like lavender, clary sage, citrus, jasmine, peppermint, and ylang-ylang diffused in the air during labor may be calming and soothing.

Make sure you try the fragrances before going to the hospital to ensure that you like them, and check with your health-care provider to be certain that your hospital allows them.

TENS MACHINE

Transcutaneous electrical nerve stimulation machine (TENS Machine) is a portable handheld device that is connected with wires to electrodes on your back.

As it activates, low-voltage electrical impulses interrupt the pain signals going to your brain, reducing pain. You control the amount and level of stimulation.

STERILE WATER INJECTIONS

A tiny amount of sterile water is injected under the skin around your lower back (sacrum) to ease lower back pain. You experience about a 30-second intense stinging sensation, which wears off, and as it does, you feel relief from back pain. The effect last for up to two hours.

PAIN RELIEF
PAIN MANAGEMENT/MEDICATED

As its name implies, medicated pain management is the use of medication to dull or eliminate pain.

MEDICATED OPTIONS

There are two types of medications:

1. Analgesic Pain Medication
Medication that lessens pain.

2. Anesthesia Pain Medication
Medication that blocks pain.

Mommy Hack

Be careful not to wait too long to take pain meds, because when the pain comes, it may take time for the medication to take effect. Be mindful and plan ahead.

MEDICATED OPTIONS

OPTIONS	PROS	CONS	EFFECT ON BABY
ANALGESICS Pain Medication: Given as an injection or through IV.	Decreased sense of contractions. Pain relief without total loss of feeling or muscle movement. Mom is awake.	Not total pain relief; just lessens it. May cause nausea, drowsiness, vomiting. May not be available an hour before delivery.	Can cause the baby to be drowsy.
EPIDURAL Local pain-blocking procedure, which injects continuous medication into the lower back through an IV.	Pain relief from the waist down. Dosage easily increased or decreased. Works for vaginal and Cesarean births. Mom can rest during long deliveries. Mom is awake and alert.	Takes about 20 min. to do and about 10–20 mins to take effect. Can increase the length of labor. Mom will not be able to use legs or move around. Lowers blood pressure.	Usually none. If Mom's blood pressure drops, baby's heartbeat can be affected.

NOTE: The information provided is not a substitute for professional medical advice, diagnosis, or treatment. Always consult your obstetrician or primary health-care provider to ensure that a treatment or medication is right and safe for you and your baby.

MEDICATED OPTIONS

OPTIONS	PROS	CONS	EFFECT ON BABY
SPINAL BLOCK Medication is injected into the fluid below the spinal cord in lower back.	Mom is awake. Takes effect right away. Complete pain relief for lower body. Lasts for one to two hours.	Can decrease your blood pressure. You might develop fever or itchiness or soreness in your back.	Might affect baby's heartbeat if Mom's blood pressure drops.
COMBINED SPINAL BLOCK & EPIDURAL	Benefits of both.	Drawbacks of both.	Effects of both.
NITROUS OXIDE A gas that is inhaled. Self-administered via a mask.	Quick, easy, and safe. Can be easily started and discontinued. No effect on labor or contractions. Mom is alert and able to move around.	Can cause drowsiness, light-headedness in some. Does not eliminate pain for all women. Might cause nausea, vomiting, or dizziness.	No significant adverse effect on baby.
LOCAL ANESTHETIC Injection of a numbing agent.	Mom is awake. Pain blocking for the episiotomy. No negative effects.	Doesn't relieve labor pain. Allergic reaction possible.	None.
GENERAL ANESTHESIA An IV makes Mom completely asleep. Usually for emergency.	Mom is not awake. Mom feels no pain.	Mom is asleep for birth. Can cause nausea and vomiting after waking.	Baby may be drowsy, requiring help breathing after birth.
TRANQUILIZERS Usually used along with analgesics to relax, and eases anxiety.	Mom is awake.	High risk of side effects.	Can negatively affect baby.
OPIOIDS Lessens pain. Injected or through IV.	Takes effect quickly.	Doesn't completely eliminate pain. Can cause nausea, vomiting, and drowsiness.	May cause baby to be drowsy and affect baby's breathing.

BUYING A BREAST PUMP

WHAT TO KNOW

Deciding on a breast pump can be confusing. They are actually very specific to each woman's situation and, unfortunately, there is no way to know ahead of time what your milk supply is going to be and how you will respond to a given pump.

WHAT IS IT?

BREAST PUMP: This device attaches to your breast and extracts milk using suction. It is used to maintain or increase your milk supply and also to relieve engorged breasts or blocked milk ducts.

TYPES OF PUMPS

- Manual pumps
- Battery-powered pumps
- Electric pumps
- Single-breast pumps
- Double-breast pumps
- Wearable, hands-free pumps

CONSIDERATIONS

- Price
- Strength
- Speed
- Comfort
- What pump insurance covers
- Noise
- Portability
- Open or closed system

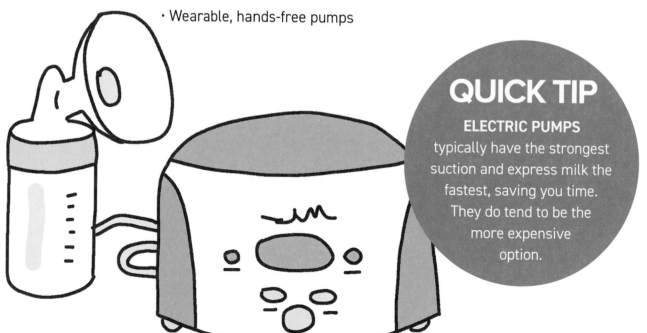

QUICK TIP

ELECTRIC PUMPS typically have the strongest suction and express milk the fastest, saving you time. They do tend to be the more expensive option.

ELECTRIC PUMP OPTIONS

RENTAL PUMPS

- Have hospital-grade motors that will pump more milk in less time.

- Quieter.

- Can help increase your supply.

- Can be helpful when pumping for several babies, a preemie, or a baby who is having difficulty breastfeeding.

- Somewhat bulky and heavy.

- Cost about $50 per month.

- Can be easily returned if pumping doesn't work for you.

PURCHASED PUMPS

- $50 for a hand pump.
  $250–$400 for a high-quality pump.
  $1,000 for a hospital-grade pump.
  $400–$500 for a wearable pump.

- If you plan on pumping for a longer period of time, or you plan on using it for several children, it might be a wiser investment.

- Lightweight and easy to carry.

- Better for only occasional pumping.

ADDITIONAL THINGS TO CONSIDER

DON'T BUY OR BORROW SOMEONE ELSE'S PUMP:

Because of the risk of cross-contamination, it is best not to borrow a pump or use a secondhand pump. (Hospital-grade rentals are built with protective barriers and approved by the FDA for multiple users.)

INSURANCE:

Check your insurance policy: it may pay for some of the pump rental or purchase cost, especially if you or your baby has a condition that makes breastfeeding difficult.

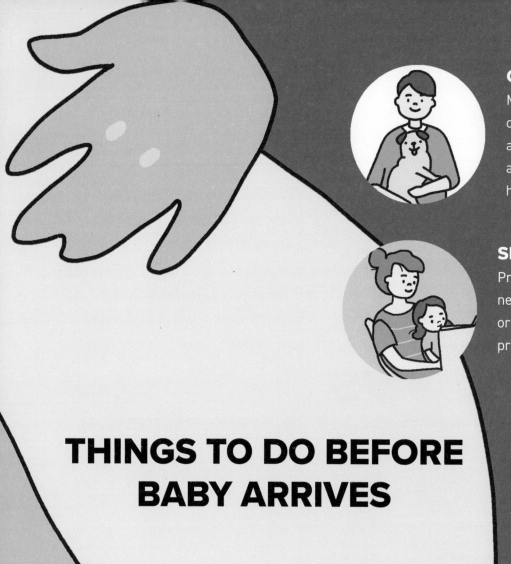

THINGS TO DO BEFORE BABY ARRIVES

CHILD & PET CARE
Make arrangements for other children or pets as far as who will look after them at a moment's notice if you have to rush to the hospital.

SIBLINGS
Prepare the siblings for the new baby by reading stories or getting them to help with preparation for the baby.

PICK A NAME
It's time to research and pick a name for your little one, so you have it ready for the birth certificate.

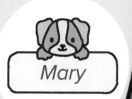

Mary

GET GEARED UP
Get any essential baby gear, stroller, car seat, etc., and install or assemble them so they are ready when you are.

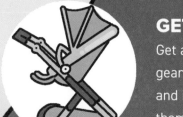

DOCUMENTS

Finish your birth plan and give copies to your health-care team. Complete any medical forms needed, update your will, and preregister at the hospital.

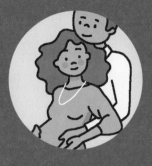

BABYMOON

Take a mini vacation before baby arrives, as extra time will be in VERY short supply after delivery.

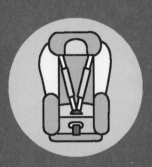

INSTALL CAR SEAT

Have your baby car seat; install it ahead of time—that first time is always more complicated than you think it will be.

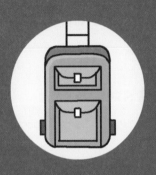

PREPARE FOR DELIVERY

Prepare for the delivery, take prenatal class(es), prepack your bag, plan the best routes, where to park, and how long you can park there.

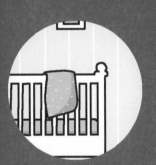

FINISH NURSERY

Complete the nursery, and have everything you need for bathing, dressing, feeding, and caring for baby.

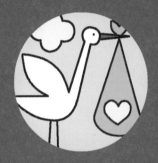

ANNOUNCEMENT

Decide on a design for the birth announcement, have a mailing list and stamps ready, and if you plan on using a photographer, book them now.

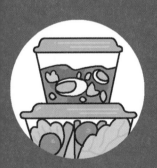

PREPARE MEALS!

Make extra meals and freeze them for easy-to-reheat eats. Stock up the pantry and fridge for whole family. Look into grocery delivery options.

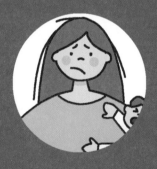

POSTPARTUM

Have postpartum supplies ready: pads, peri bottle, Tucks, medications, etc.

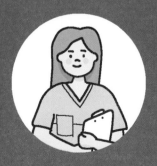

CARE

Take care of your health needs—your dentist, eye doctor, etc., and fill any needed prescriptions. Choose a pediatrician and find child care.

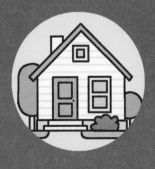

PREPARE HOUSE

Clean and prep the house for baby and guests. Finish any house projects. Start thinking about childproofing.

PREPARING THE NURSERY

NOW FOR SOME FUN

You are well on your way to becoming a new mommy or daddy, so it's time to talk nursery.

QUICK TIP

When to start the nursery?

Beginning around:
WEEK 21

Completed by:
WEEK 35

DETERMINE THE SPACE

Figure out where you want the nursery to be.

FIND YOUR STYLE

What do you want the nursery to look like? You may have a single item (a picture, a piece of furniture, or a clip of wallpaper) that can be the inspiration for everything else. If not, you may find it helpful to jump online and scroll various styles until you find one you like.

BE PRACTICAL

Plan your space to work for the activities that will be taking place in it. You'll need areas for sleeping, changing diapers, playing, and feeding your baby. So, keep in mind that you are going to need functional furniture and pieces to do those things.

FOUR MAIN PIECES OF FURNITURE

Crib

A sturdy crib with the space between slats no larger than 2 3/8 inches apart.

Chair

A comfortable rocker or glider with no exposed, moving parts or gaps that could trap or pinch fingers.

Dresser/Changing Table

A sturdy dresser with several drawers, or a long, low dresser that a changing pad can be secured to.

Lights

Lighting in the room that can be dimmed at night during changes and feeding.

DESIGN TO GROW

Choose items that allow flexibility, so that when your baby grows, you don't have to make major changes. Select furniture and pieces that can transition easily from a nursery to an older child's room.

STORAGE

It's surprising how much room babies' and children's stuff takes up. Be sure to make choices that provide for those storage needs.

DRESSER VS. CHANGING TABLE

Both can be good options if you take certain things into account.

If a changing table: Be sure that the changing area top can be removed so that when your baby grows, you are not stuck with a non-functioning piece.

If a dresser: Be sure that it's wide and long enough to fit a changing pad.

BUDGET

Determine a budget so you can plan for what things are priorities and what might be items that you can do without or work around.

GET YOUR <u>FREE</u> NURSERY ESSENTIALS LIST:

Scan the QR code for our printable essentials checklist of everything you will need for your nursery.

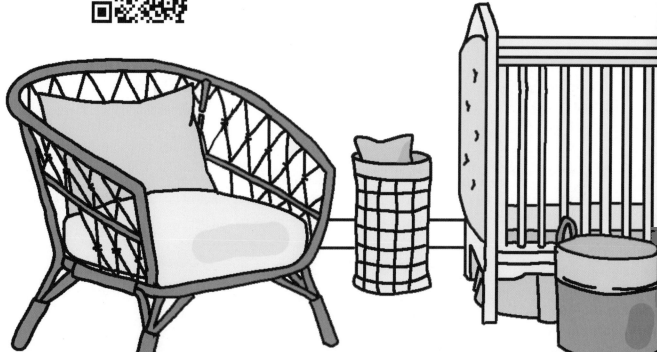

THE MUST-HAVES
FOR THE NURSERY

GET THE RIGHT STUFF!

Scan the QR code to get our recommendations for the best nursery products and essential items so you save money and time.

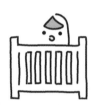

1 CRIB

The crib should be sturdy and have fixed sides. The space between the slats should be no more than 2 3/8 inches apart. The headboard should be solid with no decorative cutouts or post embellishments that a child's clothing could get caught on. Look for a crib made of ecofriendly, sustainable materials and nontoxic paint.

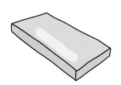

1 MATTRESS

Look for a firm, Greenguard-certified mattress about six inches deep. It should be hypoallergenic and free of phthalates, lead, and mercury. It should fit snugly in the crib with no space between the mattress and the crib sides.

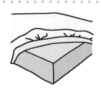

2 WATERPROOF MATTRESS COVERS

Look for a fitted, waterproof cover that is breathable and hypoallergenic.

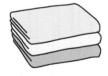

2 TO 3 FITTED SHEETS

100 percent organic fitted crib sheets made of fabrics that are either woven cottons, cotton blends, or lightweight flannel.

1 SMOKE DETECTOR

A smoke detector should be inside every sleeping room in your home, including the nursery.

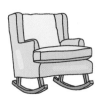

1 CHAIR

Look for a sturdy, comfortable rocker or glider with wide, padded armrests and good back support. Make sure there are no exposed, moving parts or gaps in the structure that could trap or pinch fingers. The ability to swivel and recline are pluses.

1 CARBON MONOXIDE DETECTOR

This device detects carbon monoxide (CO) gas, which is poisonous.

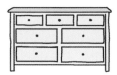

1 DRESSER

Choose a sturdy dresser with several drawers. We recommend a long, low dresser so you can secure a changing pad to the top of it and avoid purchasing a separate changing table.

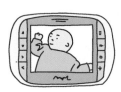

1 BABY MONITOR

Choose a video or wireless monitor that can be recharged or plugged into an outlet. One with night vision provides a clearer image when the lights are low or off. It should have the ability to zoom in and turn so when your baby moves, it can follow it. One with the ability to monitor the room temperature is a plus.

1 LAUNDRY HAMPER

You will need a laundry hamper for all the many dirty clothes, bibs, sheets, burp cloths, etc.

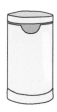

1 DIAPER PAIL

Choose a tall, waterproof pail with good capacity that has a filter or some other device for odor control. Look for a pail that opens with a foot pedal.

CORD BLOOD & TISSUE BANK

Cord blood and tissue banking is the process of saving the remaining blood in the umbilical cord or cord tissue for potential future use.

WHAT IS CORD BLOOD BANKING?

It is the collection and storage of blood from the umbilical cord at birth. The umbilical cord blood contains blood-forming stem cells, which are potentially useful for treating conditions of the blood and immune system.

The fluid is easy to collect and has more stem cells than those collected from bone marrow.

If an immediate family member has a disease that requires a bone marrow transplant, cord blood from a newborn child may have the potential to be a treatment for the genetic parents and the siblings.

QUICK TIP

You will need to order the blood-banking kit ahead of time, and let your doctor and hospital know before the birth that you are banking the blood or tissue.

TYPES OF CORD BLOOD BANKS

Public Banking

Organizations that store donated cord blood for other sick children and research. This blood is available to anyone.

Private Banking

Cord blood banks that store your baby's cord blood for your family for an annual fee.

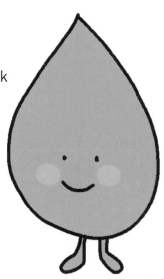

WHAT IS CORD TISSUE BANKING?

This process preserves a segment of your baby's umbilical cord, which can contain millions of stem cells of various kinds that can develop into tissue to form the nervous system, sensory organs, circulatory tissues, skin, bone, and cartilage.

These cells can be preserved for future use to potentially treat diseases and medical conditions.

WHAT TO KNOW

If you are interested in banking either cord blood and/or tissue, you will need to plan ahead to do this.

Currently, cord blood and tissue banking isn't routine in hospital or home deliveries. You will need to notify your doctor and hospital before the birth that you are interested in banking.

You will also need to obtain the cord blood kit, which you must order ahead of time from the cord blood bank you have chosen, so that you can bring it to the hospital when you go in for delivery.

Once the blood/tissue is collected, you will need to notify the bank that it is ready for pickup and transport to the bank.

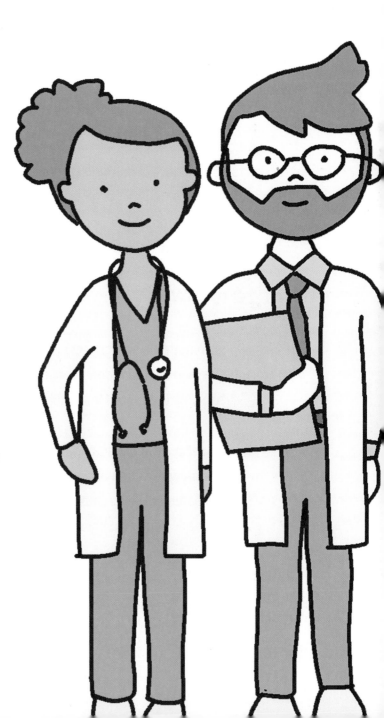

WAX ON, WAX OFF?
PREPARING YOUR PRIVATES

Mommy Hack

If you are trimming your privates yourself, consider using an electric razor with a shield to prevent any painful nicks and cuts.

The idea of having a whole crew of people between your legs checking out what is going on down there, well, it can be a bit weird and embarrassing. Waxing, shaving, trimming, or going au natural—what is a girl to do?

HAIR

During pregnancy, your hair will grow faster and in places you would prefer it didn't.

That said, self-care/grooming can take on a whole new life, especially when you are balancing a bowling ball on your stomach.

Fortunately, things will return to normal about six months after delivery. In the meantime, here are the things you need to know about safely removing hair.

WHAT TO KNOW

EMBARRASSED: You might be self-conscious about exposing it all, but the truth is doctors and the medical team don't concern themselves with your grooming techniques; they are only interested in having a safe delivery for you and your baby.

SHAVING: You should avoid shaving your privates beyond 36 weeks of pregnancy, as shaving can result in micro-cuts to the skin. These tiny nicks create potential risks of infection whether you are delivering vaginally or having a C-section.

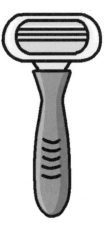

PERSONAL: PREFERENCE Whether you feel comfortable with groomed privates or not is completely up to you.

DOCTOR'S: CHOICE If the doctor decides it is necessary, they will shave you during delivery.

TIPS FOR PREPPING YOUR PRIVATES, IF YOU WANT TO

SHAVING:
AVOID beyond 36 weeks because of risk of infection.

TRIMMING:
Using trimming scissors is perfectly safe and clean; just be careful not to nick or cut yourself.

ELECTRIC SHAVERS:
Perfectly fine to maintain tidiness.

BIKINI WAX:
Considered less harmful than shaving. May cause some sensitivity.

BRAZILIAN WAX:
Considered less harmful than shaving. Be sure to let the aesthetician know you are pregnant. May cause some skin sensitivity.

SUGARING:
Considered less harmful than shaving as it rarely causes micro-cuts. You might need help from a professional.

HAIR REMOVAL CREAMS:
Considered safe, but since they contain chemicals, we suggest you consult with your health-care provider or avoid using them.

FALSE LABOR
JUST KIDDING

WHAT IS IT?

FALSE LABOR (also known as **Braxton-Hicks Contractions**):

Contractions that come and go without any pattern or consistency. It is not true labor. It's your body's way of practicing for real labor, but unlike real contractions, these don't change the shape of the cervix.

WHEN DOES IT HAPPEN?

Typically, false labor happens in the third trimester, around the last two to four weeks before your due date. Although less common, they can occur as early as the second trimester.

FALSE LABOR
TYPICALLY OCCURS
2-4 WEEKS
BEFORE YOUR DUE DATE

WHAT IS IT LIKE?

False labor can last from thirty seconds up to two minutes. It may feel like a tightening in the abdomen that comes and goes, sort of like tightening and then loosening a belt around your abdomen. They have been described as feeling like mild menstrual cramps.

TRIGGERS

Certain things can set off false labor:

- Especially active adult or baby
- Excessive pressure on the uterus

NOTE: If you have any questions or concerns, contact your health-care provider, especially if you are leaking fluid, notice a decrease in fetal movement, or are bleeding.

HOW TO TELL THE DIFFERENCE

	FALSE LABOR	TRUE LABOR
HOW OFTEN	• Irregular • No regular pattern	• Rhythmic • Once started, they continue in frequency.
HOW STRONG	• Varying intensity	• Progressively get stronger.
DO THEY CHANGE	• They may stop or weaken if you start to move, walk, or change position.	• Continue regardless of movement or change in position.
PAINS LOCATION	• Felt in the front of the body.	• Starts in the back, moves to the front of your body.
SIGNS OF LABOR	• Cervix does NOT open.	• Cervix thins and opens. • Vaginal discharge BROWNISH, PINK, REDDISH • Possible nausea, vomiting • Possible rise in blood pressure • Mucus plug

ITS TRUE LABOR IF

5-1-1 RULE:

• Contractions come every five minutes.
• Lasting about one minute each.
• For about one hour or more.

MUCUS PLUG
POPPING THE CORK

Anything coming out of your body can make you anxious and stressed, but expelling this plug is a normal part of all pregnancies and a potentially exciting sign that baby will soon be on its way.

WHAT IS IT?

MUCUS PLUG: Functions like a seal in the cervix that creates a barrier to the uterus. It's made up of mucus that accumulates in the cervix.

WHAT DOES IT DO?

Its purpose is to protect the baby during pregnancy from bacteria and infections by preventing them from entering the uterus.

WHAT'S IT LIKE?

· Clear, off-white, pinkish, red, or brownish in color

· A thick, sticky, jelly-like substance

· Stringy texture

· Around one to two inches long

· Rather odorless

The discharge can be as thick as one string, one big glob, or small segments.

WHEN DOES IT HAPPEN?

The discharge of the mucus plug is a normal part of the birthing process; it occurs when you are nearing the end of your pregnancy.

It can mean several things:

1. You are approaching labor (may be days or a couple weeks away).
2. It may be the beginning of labor.

In many cases, contractions will start soon after losing the mucus plug.

NOTE: Every pregnancy is different, so speak to your health-care provider if you lose your mucus plug and have any questions or concerns.

THE MUCUS PLUG

WHAT TO DO

First, stay calm. If you are full-term, determine if you are having frequent contractions; if so, contact your health-care provider. If not, wait until you are. Labor is usually a slow buildup.

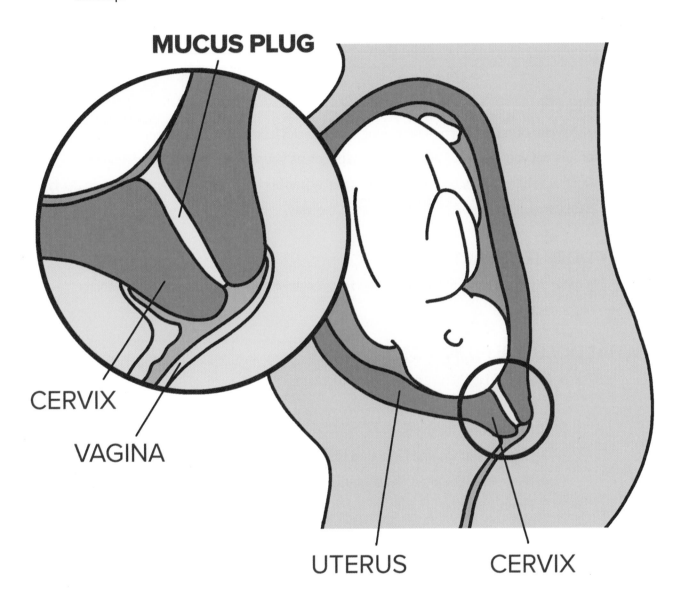

MUCUS PLUG

CERVIX

VAGINA

UTERUS

CERVIX

WHEN TO CALL THE DOC
Contact your doctor if:

- You experience bleeding, like a menstrual period.
- If you notice something that looks like your mucus plug discharged before 37 weeks.

WATER BREAKING

GETTING STARTED

This can be scary and exciting all at the same time; it signals that your baby will be coming soon.

QUICK TIP

Have a doggy pee pad or a towel in your cars in case your water breaks en route or to catch any leaks after your water breaks.

WHAT IS IT?

The water-filled sac surrounding your baby breaks (rupture of membranes, ROM) and drains out your vagina. This naturally happens as your body prepares for delivery. Contractions typically begin soon after your water breaks, but there can be a slight delay; either way, it's a sign that your baby is on the way.

WHY DOES IT BREAK?

It naturally occurs when the baby's head moves down the birth canal or as the result of contractions.

WHAT DOES THE FLUID DO?

The amniotic fluid in the sac has several functions:

1. Cushions and protects the baby.
2. Makes room for the baby.
3. Helps the lungs and digestive system develop.
4. Keeps the temperature constant.
5. Fights infection.

WHAT'S YOUR WATER BREAKING LIKE?

Every woman experiences her water breaking differently. It could be a slow trickle or a rapid gush of water (like you peed in your pants). You might experience pain, cramps, and contractions.

- It's usually clear or pale yellow.
- Odorless or slightly sweet smelling.
- Can be about four cups' worth of fluid.

MY WATER JUST BROKE; WHAT TO DO?

STAY CALM

Don't panic.

CALL YOUR HEALTH-CARE PROVIDER

Your doctor, midwife, or nurse may advise you to stay home and see if your contractions start, or they might want you to come in to examine you.

TIME YOUR CONTRACTIONS

You may be asked to time your contractions as you wait for your labor to progress.

WEAR A PAD

Consider wearing a pad or panty liner to catch leakage, but DO NOT use a tampon.

NIMBLE

You can eat during early labor, and you might want to consider doing so because, once you are admitted to the hospital, you may not be able to eat anything.

RELAX

If you are waiting for labor to progress, try to relax and rest.

Mommy Hack

Protect your mattress by putting a waterproof mattress cover on your bed just in case your water breaks in the middle of the night.

MY WATER HAS NOT BROKEN

If your water doesn't break on its own, your doctor might break it; this is called artificial rupture of membranes (AROM).

CONCERNS

· Prelabor preterm rupture of membranes (PPROM)—water breaking before 37 weeks.

NOTE:

If you are not certain your water has broken, contact your health-care provider, who can confirm if it has by performing a physical examination or ultrasound.

3RD TRIMESTER CONCERNS

WHAT TO LOOK OUT FOR

Common warning signs that could indicate a more serious issue.

OVERVIEW

You are on the home stretch, quite literally. Knowing the difference between symptoms that are normal and those that are not is important. There are some serious, late-pregnancy warning signs and symptoms that you should be aware of.

CONCERNS TO SHARE WITH YOUR DOCTOR

VAGINAL BLEEDING

Any significant bleeding can be an indication of a problem.

SEVERE VAGINAL PAIN

While cramping is not usual, any severe vaginal pain needs to be looked at.

FEVER OR CHILLS

If you experience a fever of 100.4°F and/or chills, let your doctor know.

SWELLING

If you experience sudden or severe swelling of the face, hands, or fingers, contact your doctor.

SUDDEN WEIGHT GAIN OR LOSS

If you gain more than 6.5 pounds per month or experience too little weight gain, notify your provider.

INTENSE ABDOMINAL PAIN

Any abdominal pain that is prolonged or associated with bleeding is cause for concern.

EXTREME NAUSEA OR VOMITING

Any severe vomiting that will not go away may indicate a problem.

SEVERE DIZZINESS

Any kind of dizziness or blurred vision should be reported to your doctor.

PAINFUL OR BURNING URINATION

Pain while urinating or decreased urine output could be a sign of an infection.

GESTATIONAL DIABETES

Your doctor will continue to monitor you for this condition.

HEADACHES

Headaches that will not go away with medication.

FLOATERS IN YOUR EYES

Seeing spots in your vision.

CONTRACTIONS

Contractions or tightening of the uterus before 36 weeks may indicate that labor is beginning.

VAGINAL DISCHARGE

Notify your doctor of a significant increase in vaginal discharge.

LACK OF BABY MOVEMENT

If you notice a lack of or decreased movement, let your doctor know.

WARNING

Contact your doctor immediately if you experience any of these symptoms. They will determine whether it is something serious or if it needs to be monitored.

Sometimes
the smallest things
take up the most
room in your heart.

DELIVERY

What you really need to know about and prepare before the big day arrives.

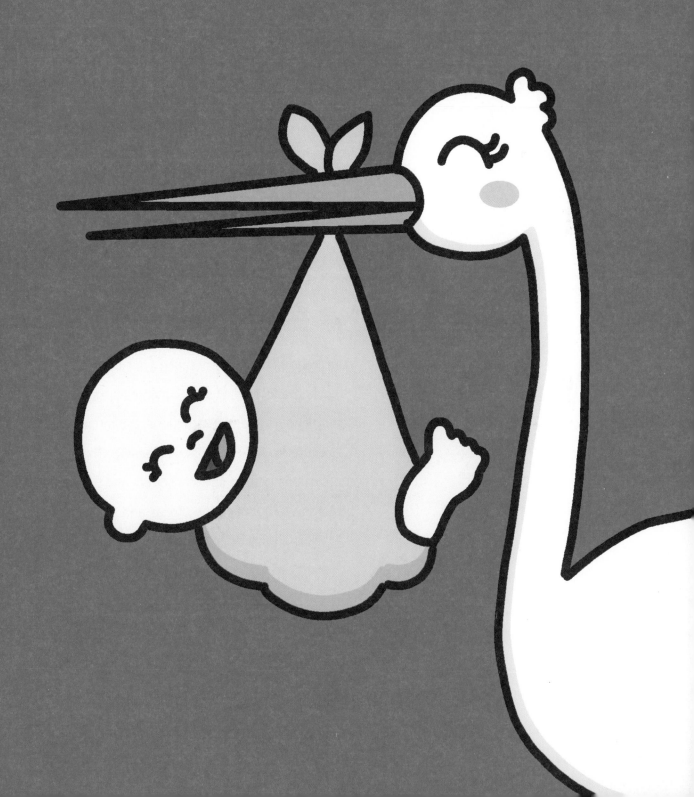

STAGES OF LABOR

OVERVIEW

Although there are specific stages in the process of having a baby, how long and how difficult each stage is varies from person to person and pregnancy to pregnancy.

STAGE

1

CONTRACTIONS

During the first stage of labor, your body begins to prepare to give birth by having increasingly strong and frequent contractions, the muscles of the uterus tightening and releasing. These contractions help to stretch, soften, and open the passageway between the uterus and the vagina. This allows the baby to move into the birth canal. Once the cervix is fully open (dilated), you will begin the next stage of labor.

DELIVERY

During this stage, your baby is born. You will feel increased pressure on your rectum, and your health-care provider will direct you when to push hard or soft or not at all. It's during this time that you might try different positions, until you find the one that is most comfortable for you. As your baby enters the world, first comes the head, followed soon after by the rest of it. The airway is cleared, and the cord is cut.

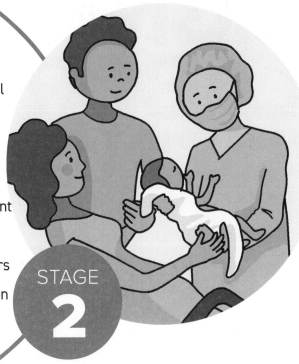

STAGE
2

AFTERBIRTH

The final stage of labor is the delivery of the placenta. This process can take between 30 minutes and an hour. During this time, you might hold your baby in your arms or the staff might rest it on you. You will continue to feel mild contractions that are closer together as the placenta is moved into the birth canal. You will be asked to push one final time to deliver the placenta.

STAGE
3

SIGNS OF LABOR
WHAT TO LOOK FOR

You are reaching your due date, and it's that time, but is it really? It's important to know the signs of labor.

WHAT IS IT?

LABOR: The body's natural process of giving birth. You are in labor when you have regular contractions that cause your cervix to change (effacement).

TIPS THAT LABOR MAY BE COMING

BABY DROPPING

The process whereby the baby settles into the pelvis—also called lightening. It means that your baby is getting into position. You might notice that you are having an easier time breathing.

NESTING INSTINCT

In the days or weeks leading up to labor, it's not usual to experience a sudden burst of energy to prepare your home. Some women and even men find themselves with a strong urge to get ready for their baby during this time.

CONTRACTIONS

Having strong, regular contractions.

VAGINAL DISCHARGE

When the cervix begins to open, the mucus plug is released; it may be clear, pink, or slightly brownish.

INCREASED BLOOD PRESSURE

Your blood pressure may rise while you are going into labor; your doctor will monitor it.

FEELINGS OF PRESSURE OR FULLNESS

You may start to feel pressure in your pelvis or vagina as the baby drops down into position for delivery; try to relax and rest.

CRAMPING AND BACK PAIN

You might begin to experience pain in your lower back.

WATER BREAKING

The rupture of the amniotic sac may occur.

NAUSEA/VOMITING

If you have a full stomach and labor begins, it is not unusual for you to experience nausea and even to vomit.

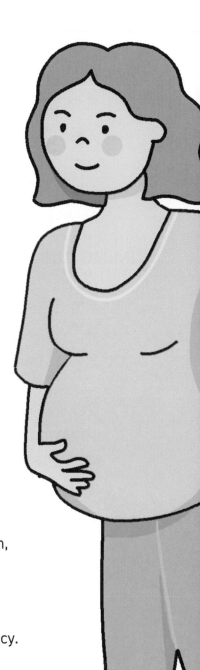

BABY'S MOVEMENT

You may notice that your baby is moving less as you near the start of labor. This may be a sign of distress; if you notice a lack of activity, let you doctor know.

DIARRHEA

As your muscles relax and loosen in preparation for the birth, other muscles relax too, including those in the rectum, which can cause diarrhea.

WEIGHT GAIN

Your weight gain often levels off at the end of your pregnancy.

CONTRACTIONS
WHAT TO KNOW

GET YOUR <u>FREE</u> CONTRACTION TRACKING CHART

Scan the QR code to get our free contraction tracking chart.

WHAT IS IT?

CONTRACTIONS: As labor begins, you will experience contractions—the periodic tightening and relaxing of the muscles of the uterus. These contractions help your baby move down and through the birth canal.

They feel like a cramping or tightening that begins in your back and moves around to the front of your body. It might feel like pressure in your back or pelvis, similar to menstrual cramps.

TIMING CONTRACTIONS

You time contractions by noting the time when:

- A contraction starts.
- A contraction stops.
- The next contraction starts.

Your doctor may ask you about the:

DURATION (the length of each contraction)

FREQUENCY (how far apart the contractions are)

Generally, your health-care providers want you to track your contractions for an hour or more.

This will help give them an indication of how far along you are in your labor and if it's time to head to the hospital.

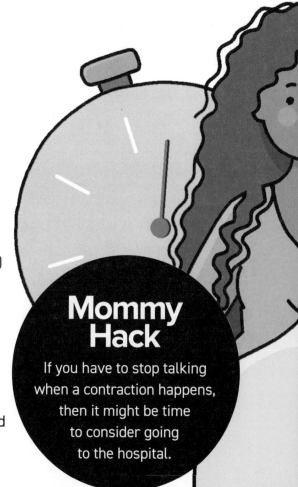

Mommy Hack

If you have to stop talking when a contraction happens, then it might be time to consider going to the hospital.

CONTRACTIONS

WHAT THE DOCTOR WILL ASK YOU

How long is each contraction (duration)?
How far apart are they (frequency)?
How long have you been feeling them?

YOU'LL GET THE ANSWERS TO THESE QUESTIONS BY USING THE BELOW.

CONTRACTION <u>START TIME</u>
CONTRACTION <u>STOP TIME</u> **=** **DURATION** OF CONTRACTION

<u>START TIME</u> OF ONE CONTRACTION
<u>START TIME</u> OF THE NEXT CONTRACTION **=** **FREQUENCY** OF CONTRACTIONS

YOU'LL TRACK YOUR CONTRACTION
FOR AT LEAST AN HOUR **=** HOW LONG HAVE YOU BEEN FEELING THEM?

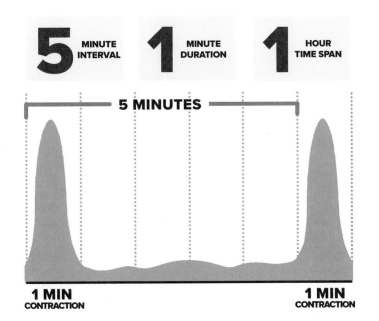

5 MINUTE INTERVAL **1** MINUTE DURATION **1** HOUR TIME SPAN

5 MINUTES

1 MIN CONTRACTION   1 MIN CONTRACTION

SO, WHEN TO GO TO THE HOSPITAL?

Typically, you will want to be ready to go to the hospital when your contractions reach the 5-1-1 Rule.

5-1-1 RULE =
- Contractions are five minutes apart.
- Each contraction lasts about one minute.
- Contractions have been tracked one hour.

INDUCING LABOR

WHAT, WHY, AND HOW

It is impossible to predict how labor and delivery will progress, and sometimes it may be necessary to help move things along.

QUICK TIP

An induced labor may make labor pains more painful than natural childbirth, as natural labor contractions build up slowly; induced labor can start more quickly and be stronger.

WHAT IS IT?

INDUCING LABOR: The process of prompting the uterus to contract and go into labor. It is done with labor-inducing medications or some other technique.

WHY DO IT?

- **Post-term pregnancy:** You are one to two weeks past your due date.
- **Rupture of amniotic sac:** Your water has broken, but labor has not begun.
- **Infection:** An infection of the uterus, placenta, or amniotic fluid occurs.
- **Fetal growth restriction:** The baby has stopped growing at the expected rate.
- **Amniotic fluid:** There is not enough amniotic fluid surrounding the baby.
- **Diabetes:** You already had or have developed diabetes.
- **High blood pressure:** You have chronic high blood pressure or gestational hypertension.
- **Medical condition:** You have heart, lung, or kidney disease or are very overweight.
- **Multiples:** You are carrying multiple babies.

CASCADE OF INTERVENTION

Inducing labor can have the unintended effect of leading to another intervention, which can lead to another, and so on. This is referred to as "cascade of intervention." You should use care in deciding to have an intervention, weighing the benefits and risks. **NOTE:** Consult your health-care provider ahead of delivery to understand all the risks.

WHY NOT DO IT?

- Previous vertical incision C-section.
- Placenta is blocking the cervix.
- Baby is not in a head-down position.
- You have active genital herpes.
- Umbilical cord is blocking the vagina.

METHODS FOR INDUCING LABOR

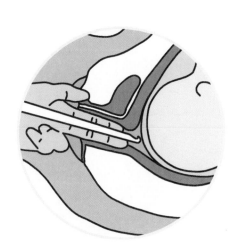

THE AMNIOTIC SAC
IS RUPTURED.

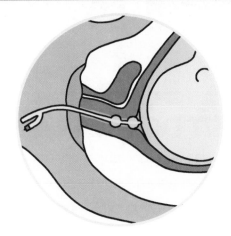

AN INFLATABLE BALLOON IS
INSERTED IN THE CERVIX AND
FILLED WITH SALINE.

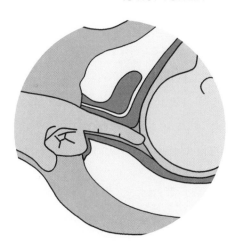

BRUSHING FINGER OVER THE
MEMBRANE COVERING
THE AMNIOTIC SAC.

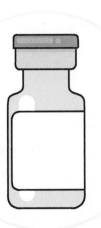

MEDICATION OR THE HORMONE
OXYTOCIN OR PROSTAGLANDINS.

NOTE: Always speak to your health-care provider about what to expect with any medical procedure to understand the risks and benefits so that you and your baby are kept safe.

POSITIONS FOR LABOR

STAND UP, SIT DOWN, PUSH-PUSH

There is no one best position for labor, and more than likely you will use several positions throughout your labor. As everyone's experiences of labor are different, you might find some positions work better for you than others.

QUICK TIP

The reclining position—lying on your back—is not an ideal position for labor. You are not working with gravity, and it can increase contraction pain.

LABOR POSITIONS

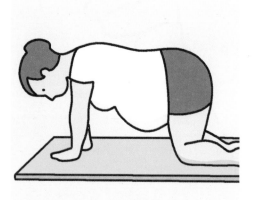

HANDS & KNEES

Being on your hands and knees is a very popular position. This position allows you to do pelvic tilts to help ease back pain. You can use this position either on a bed or on the floor. It helps to have a yoga mat to make it a bit easier on the knees and hands.

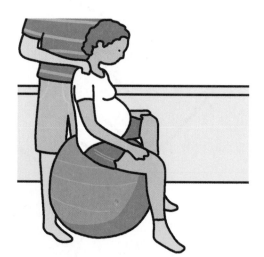

SITTING

You can sit on a chair or birthing ball with your legs apart. Try a little rocking forward and back motion to ease the pain. Sitting on a birthing ball also allows you to roll your hips. Be sure that your birth partner provides added stability.

An alternative is to straddle an armless chair or sit backward on the toilet seat. In these positions, you can lean forward, resting your arms and head to ease back strain. It also is nice to have your birth partner massage your back while in this position.

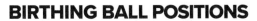

BIRTHING BALL POSITIONS

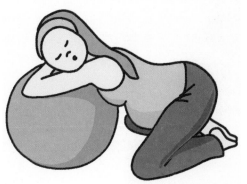

There are many positions that can be done using a birthing ball. Check out the birthing ball positions page.

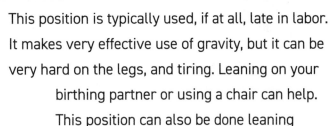

Mommy Hack

Moms emphasized: Don't be shy or nervous about asking the nurse, midwife, or hospital for whatever you want during labor!

SQUATTING

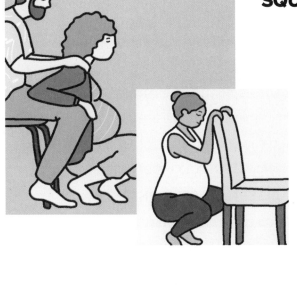

This position is typically used, if at all, late in labor. It makes very effective use of gravity, but it can be very hard on the legs, and tiring. Leaning on your birthing partner or using a chair can help. This position can also be done leaning against a wall. Be sure to have your birthing partner provide support and help getting up from this position.

LYING ON SIDE

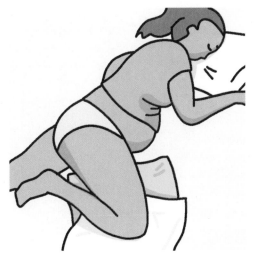

This position is especially good if you need a break from any of the other positions. In this position, your birthing partner will be able to massage your back.

Lying on your left side is best, as it allows better blood flow. Having a pillow between your legs will give added comfort.

NOTE: The information provided is not a substitute for professional medical advice, diagnosis, or treatment. Always consult your obstetrician or primary health-care provider to ensure that a treatment or medication is right and safe for you and your baby.

POSITIONS FOR LABOR
STAND UP, SIT DOWN, PUSH-PUSH-PUSH

LABOR POSITIONS CONTINUED

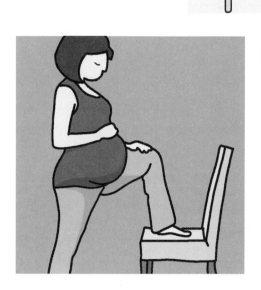

STANDING & SWAYING

Standing is a good position because it utilizes gravity. Standing in one place might be tiring, so it helps to add some movement. Some people like to dance rhythmically to their breathing or to music. You can use this position when you are alone or while leaning on your birthing partner.

ALTERNATE STANDING POSITION

You can lean on a birthing ball that is sitting on a table and rock back and forth while resting on the ball.

LUNGING

This position can be challenging and tiring, but it is very good at opening the pelvis, helping baby descend. You will want your birthing partner to provide added support.

QUICK TIP

Upright and active positions are the most effective for laboring.

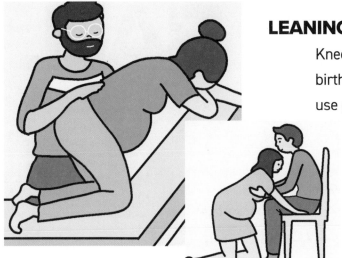

LEANING ON KNEES

Kneeling and leaning over a chair, bed, or birthing ball is a good way to ease back strain and use gravity to help your baby descend.

You can also lean on your birthing partner for greater comfort.

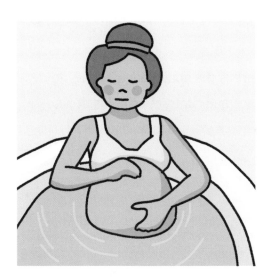

BIRTHING POOL

Some women find laboring in a pool of warm water is comforting. You can either free float or kneel in the tub.

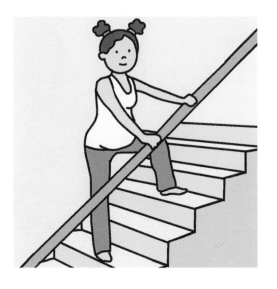

WALKING OR CLIMBING STAIRS

Some women find walking or going up and down stairs sideways helpful. During contractions, you can stop and hold onto the rail. It is very good for opening the pelvis and encouraging your baby to drop. However, it also can be very tiring over time.

NOTE: The information provided is not a substitute for professional medical advice, diagnosis, or treatment. Always consult your obstetrician or primary health-care provider to ensure that a treatment or medication is right and safe for you and your baby.

BIRTHING BALL
GETTING ON THE BALL

WHAT IS IT?

BIRTHING BALL: Slightly larger than your typical exercise ball, it is made of nonskid material. It can be used during your pregnancy to exercise or to elevate your legs to relieve back strain while you are seated. It is also used during the childbirth/labor process.

FOR LABOR

Birthing balls can be used in many labor positions. There is the added benefit of being able to sway, rock, or bounce, all of which help ease back and contraction pains. It also may help open the pelvis, allowing baby to drop more quickly and easily. It generally keeps you upright and active, which is ideal for laboring.

It's recommended you start using the birthing ball weeks or months before your labor so you are familiar with it and have practiced maintaining your balance. When using the ball during labor, have your birth partner provide added support and balance.

CHOOSING A BIRTHING BALL

Birthing balls are not one size fits all. Your knees should be four inches below your hips when you are sitting on your birthing ball.

HEIGHT	BALL SIZE
5'4" or shorter	**55 cm (21 in.)**
5'5" to 5'8"	**65 cm (26 in.)**
5'9" or taller	**75 cm (30 in.)**

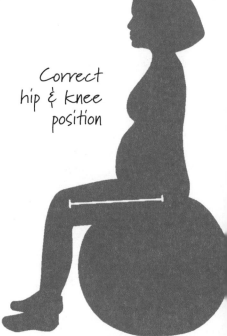

Correct hip & knee position

> ## QUICK TIP
> If your water breaks when you are using the birthing ball, it might cause the ball to skid. Be careful!

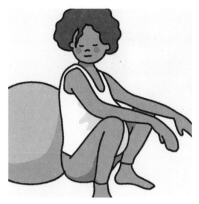

Squat and lean against the ball while it rests against the wall.

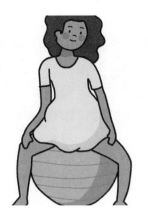

While sitting, you can bounce up and down. You can roll your hips in a circular motion or rock forward and back.

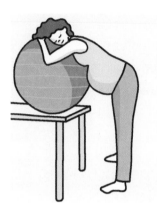

While standing, lean on the birthing ball and gently rock forward and back.

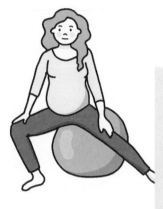

Lunge slowly from side to side while sitting on the ball.

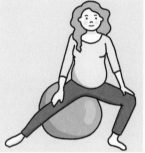

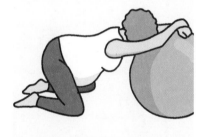

While lying on the ball, you can rock forward and back.

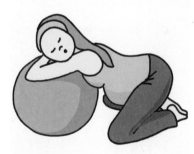

While lying on the ball, you can rock forward and back.

BIRTHING PEANUT

Similar to a birthing ball, this peanut-shaped inflatable is used by moms who have to remain in bed; for example, if they've had an epidural.

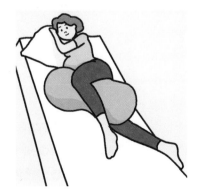

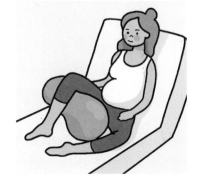

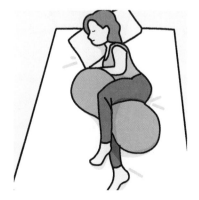

EFFACEMENT

IT'S HAPPENING NOW

As you begin the last step of labor, you will start effacement and progress to dilation. The degree of effacement and dilation will tell your health-care provider how far along you are in your labor.

WHAT IS IT?

EFFACEMENT: The process where the cervix gets ready to deliver your baby. As you go into labor and begin having contractions, the cervix starts to thin, softens, and shortens—this process is called effacement.

The degree that the cervix is effaced is measured in percentages—from 0 to 100 percent— 100 percent being fully effaced.

EFFACEMENT

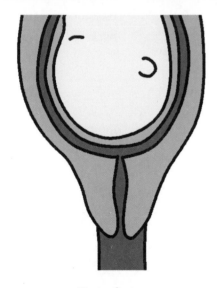

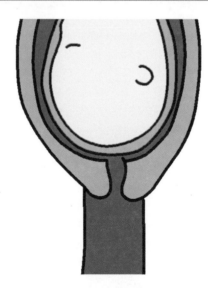

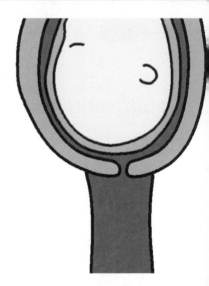

Cervix not effaced or dilated

Cervix 50% effaced and not dilated

Cervix fully effaced and 1 cm dilated

WHAT IS IT?

DILATION: The term used to describe the opening or widening of the cervix.

This is measured in centimeters—from 0 to 10—
10 centimeters being fully dilated.

YOU ARE READY FOR DELIVERY:

When you are
100% effaced and
10 centimeters dilated,

baby is on the way and moves into the birth canal.

DILATION

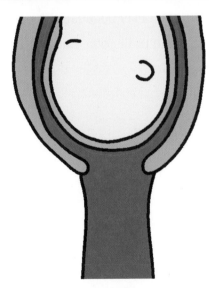

**Cervix
7 cm dilated**

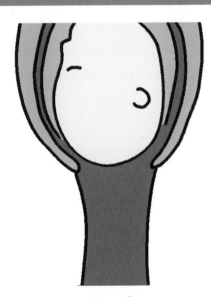

**Cervix
10 cm dilated**

HOLY CRAP!
PLEASE SAY THAT JUST DIDN'T HAPPEN

If giving birth isn't hard enough to deal with, the truth is there are a couple of unexpected and embarrassing things that are likely to happen while giving birth.

POOPING

Yes, it can and does happen often—it's perfectly NORMAL! Your health-care team has seen it before and will clean things up quickly without saying a word. The truth is that your poo tells the health-care team that you are actually pushing correctly and labor is progressing normally.

I know it's embarrassing, but it can't be helped; so forget about it, you have a baby to deliver.

PEEING

Losing control of your bladder is another embarrassing thing that also might happen. This too is completely NORMAL! It happens primarily because the pelvic floor muscles are stretched out. You may also leak for a while until your muscles tighten back up (all the more reason to do those Kegel exercises).

Those of you who have an epidural can expect that you might pee because you will lose the ability to feel whether or not your bladder is full.

TOOTING

Oh yes—toot, toot, toot away. You will fart before giving birth and more than likely during delivery too. It's NORMAL; everyone does it.

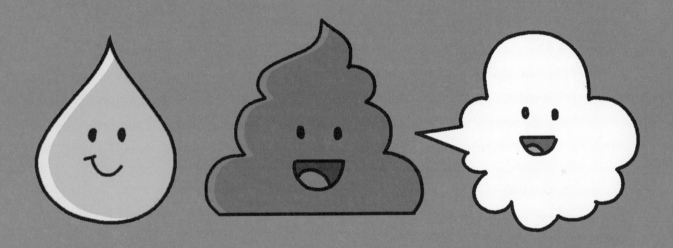

Mommy Hack

Yes—it's a thing.
Moms advise: forget about it!
Your delivery professionals
have seen it all, and
it will not phase them
in the least.

PERINEAL LACERATION

YIKES!

There is really no other way to describe a perineal laceration than to say it is a tear of the skin caused by something quite large (your baby) being pushed through a smaller opening (your vagina). Yes, the thought of it sucks, but some delivery trauma is unfortunately common.

WHAT IS IT?

PERINEAL LACERATION: Also called vaginal tearing, it is an injury to the tissue around your vagina and rectum caused by childbirth. During a vaginal delivery, the skin around the vagina thins in preparation for childbirth, when it is intended to stretch to allow your baby to pass through. But sometimes, in the process, it tears.

WHY DOES IT HAPPEN?

1. Baby is too large (eight or more pounds).

2. Delivery happens very quickly and there isn't enough time for the skin to stretch.

3. A forceps or vacuum is used during delivery.

4. It's your first delivery.

5. The baby's position: face-up delivery

6. An episiotomy.

GRADES OF TEARS

There are several grades of tears:

FIRST-DEGREE TEAR: The least severe of tears, it involves the tissue of the vagina and perineal area.

SECOND-DEGREE TEAR: The most common level of tear. This tear goes deeper into the muscle of the vagina and perineum.

THIRD-DEGREE TEAR: This tear extends from the vagina to the anus. It involves the tearing of both the tissue and the vaginal muscle and sphincter muscle, which controls bowel movements.

FOURTH-DEGREE TEAR: This tear goes from the vagina to the anus and into the rectum itself; it is the most severe of tears.

TIPS FOR PREVENTING TEARS

Unfortunately, while there are no guarantees that any method will prevent perineal tearing, minimizing the severity of tearing might be possible. Here are some methods that have been utilized:

LATERAL OR UPRIGHT POSITION:
Certain birthing positions may lower perineal trauma. Upright positions and side-lying positions appear to lower the risk of perineal trauma when compared with lying flat.

WARM COMPRESSES:
When applied to the perineum area during labor, compresses may reduce the risk of third- and fourth-degree tears.

PERINEAL MASSAGE:
Perineal massage during labor may reduce the degree of perineal trauma.

WATER BIRTHS:
Water births may help lower the risk of perineal tearing.

PUSHING AT THE RIGHT TIMES:
Waiting to push until you feel the urge to push has resulted in fewer tears. Stop pushing when the baby begins to crown to give the perineum time to stretch.

EPISIOTOMY
WHAT TO KNOW

The percentage of episiotomies varies greatly, but the number appears to be dropping. Still, it is important to understand what it is and speak to your health-care provider about their thoughts.

WHAT IS IT?

EPISIOTOMY: A surgical procedure where a cut is made to the perineum during delivery to widen the vaginal opening to help get the baby out. Episiotomies are usually avoided unless the physician needs to delivery the baby rapidly or the baby's shoulder is stuck behind the pelvic bone.

HOW IS IT DONE?

An incision is made either at the midline or laterally in the skin area between the vagina and anus (called the perineum).

WHY IS IT DONE?

Your health-care provider might recommend an episiotomy if your baby needs to be quickly delivered.

Reasons to have this procedure:

- Baby's shoulder is stuck behind the pelvic bone.
- Baby has an irregular heartbeat.
- An operative procedure is needed (like using a forceps or vacuum).
- Baby is larger than normal.

TYPES OF EPISIOTOMIES

The two most common episiotomies are:

MIDLINE EPISIOTOMY: Commonly used in North America, it is a cut which runs straight from the vagina to just above the anus.

MEDIOLATERAL: Commonly used in Europe, it is a cut which runs diagonally from the vagina—usually at a 45° angle—to the anus.

NOTE: Always speak to your health-care provider about all medical advice and procedures to understand the risks and benefits so that you and your baby are kept safe.

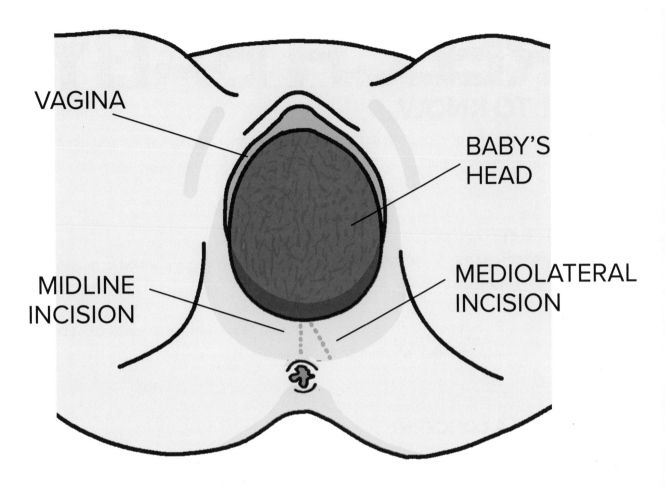

VAGINA

BABY'S
HEAD

MIDLINE
INCISION

MEDIOLATERAL
INCISION

TIPS TO PREVENT AN EPISIOTOMY

1. Try different positions during labor; that puts less stress on the perineum.

2. Understand when and how hard to push so you don't damage tissue by pushing at the wrong time.

3. With a hot, moist cloth, apply pressure to your perineum when baby's head crowns.

4. Use perineal massage to prepare the skin for stretching during delivery.

RECOVERY

Usually repaired within an hour of delivery. Sutures close the wound and will naturally dissolve in one month. You will be told to avoid certain activities during recovery. You should be fully healed in four to six weeks unless you had a severe tear.

BREECH BABY
WHAT TO KNOW

You are nearing the end of your pregnancy and the finish line is in sight when you learn that you baby is breech—now what?

WHAT IS IT?

BREECH BABY: Occurs when the baby's feet or butt is in a position to be delivered before its head is delivered.

Breech positions are more common in babies delivered early; most babies move into a head-down position by 36 weeks.

WHY IS IT A CONCERN?

There are greater risks to the baby when it is delivered in a breech position. The risks include:

- Fractures to the baby's bones.
- Problems getting the baby out.
- Dislocation of the baby's arms or legs.
- Compressed umbilical cord, which can cause nerve or brain damage.

A BREECH DELIVERY

If your baby is in a breech position, your options are to:

- Try turning baby in the womb so that baby is head first.
- Have a C-section.
- Attempt a vaginal breech delivery—this comes with increased risk.

TURNING A BABY

See the next page for tips on how to potentially turn your baby.

TYPES OF BREECH POSITIONS

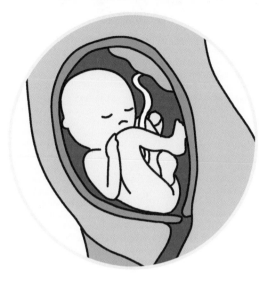

COMPLETE

When baby's butt is pointed down
and legs are folded beneath it.

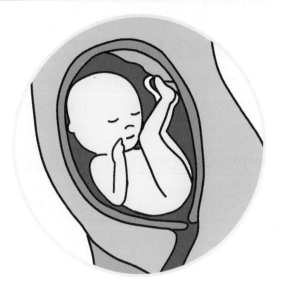

FRANK

When baby's butt is pointed down
and legs are pointed up.

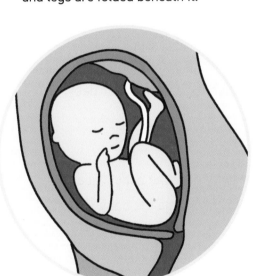

FOOTLING

When baby's butt is pointed
down and one or both legs
are pointed down
and will deliver first.

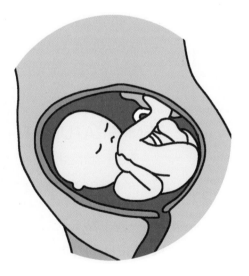

TRANSVERSE

When baby is lying sideways
across the uterus.

NOTE: The information provided is not a substitute for professional medical advice, diagnosis, or treatment. Always consult your obstetrician
or primary health-care provider to ensure that a treatment or medication is right and safe for you and your baby.

BREECH BABY
TURNING THINGS AROUND

Most babies naturally turn to a head-down position by 36 weeks, but some don't. There are several techniques used to try and get things turned around.

OPTIONS FOR TURNING BABY

Medical Procedure

1. EXTERNAL CEPHALIC VERSION:

This is a medical procedure where your health-care provider attempts to turn the baby into a head-down position by applying pressure to your stomach to manipulate your baby's position.

The procedure is typically performed at the hospital—in case any complications arise—at around 37 weeks. Women must have had a healthy pregnancy and a normal amount of amniotic fluid. If you are contemplating this procedure, consult your health-care provider to understand the risks involved and to discuss whether or not it is an option for you and your baby.

Nonmedical Procedure

2. TEMPERATURE TECHNIQUE:

Place something cold at the top of your belly near the baby's head and something warm below your belly to encourage the baby to turn.

Chiropractic Procedure

3. WEBER TECHNIQUE:

With this chiropractic procedure, the body is adjusted in an attempt to reduce the tension in your pelvis and hips and to relax your uterus to encourage your baby to turn.

Nonmedical Procedure

4. ACUPUNCTURE:

This involves placing needles at pressure points to balance the body's energy to relax the uterus and promote baby to move.

Nonmedical Procedure

5. MUSIC:

Some women have placed headphones or a speaker below their bellies to encourage their baby to turn toward the music or a recording of their voice.

Nonmedical Procedure

6. PRENATAL YOGA:

Always check with your doctor first to ensure that any poses are safe for you and your baby.

Some women have found certain modified yoga poses helped encourage baby to turn. The idea is it creates more space and aligns baby to move into position.

COMMON BREECH TURNING POSES:

- Dolphin Pose
- Child's Pose
- Downward Dog
- Cat-Cow
- Supported Bridge Pose

These poses can be difficult to do while pregnant and should be done so with assistance. If you have blood-pressure issues, you should avoid all inversion positions. If you feel lightheaded or unwell, lower yourself and roll to your left side and rest.

MODIFIED CHILD'S POSE

On your hands and knees, knees wide apart, slowly lower yourself while stretching your arms out in front of you; your butt and hips will be higher than chest.

QUICK TIP

The supported bridge pose is best done on an empty stomach to reduce acid reflux. Also make sure you have someone to support you.

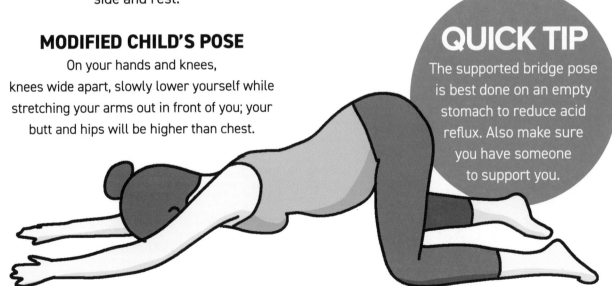

NOTE: Always speak to your health-care provider before attempting any medical or nonmedical procedures to try and turn a breech baby to ensure that it is safe for both you and baby.

BIRTHING POSITIONS
BABY IS COMING

QUICK TIP

Delivering in a more upright position rather than lying flat during delivery might reduce the risk of vaginal tearing.

There are several possible positions for giving birth; speak to your health-care provider to help determine which are most comfortable and safe for you.

WHAT IS IT?

BIRTHING POSITIONS: The position one takes when delivering a baby.

There are several types of birthing positions. Depending on where you are giving birth, if you have an epidural, or if there are complications, not all positions may be allowed; check with your health-care team.

COMMON BIRTHING POSITIONS

POSITION 1: **SQUATTING**

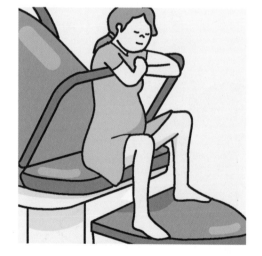

Squatting is one of the most effective birthing positions. The squatting position helps expand the pelvis, giving more room and good alignment for baby to move through the birth canal. It also works with gravity to help bring baby down and out.

The position should be done with the aid of a doula, a partner, or a birthing bar. A birthing bar is a device that attaches to the bed that helps support the mom while she is sitting or squatting. You can sit while in between contractions to rest and then move into a squat during the contraction.

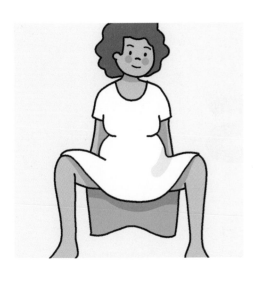

POSITION 2: **SITTING**

This position typically utilizes a low stool (birthing stool) that is shaped a bit like a toilet. This position maintains an upright position that works with gravity to help bring the baby down and out.

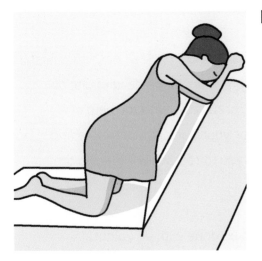

POSITION 3: **KNEELING**

The kneeling position can be especially helpful for women experiencing back pain. During contractions you can squat down on your knees while pushing and then raise back up and lean on the bed to rest. You can also kneel while using a birthing bar or birthing ball. An alternative position is to kneel on one knee, while placing your other foot flat on the bed.

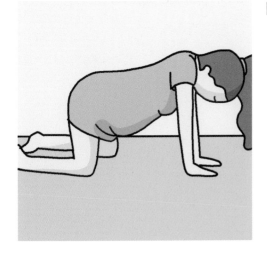

POSITION 4: **HANDS AND KNEES**

Also called doggie style, this popular position allows you to do pelvic tilts and helps ease back pain. You can do this position either on a bed or on the floor. It helps to have a yoga mat to ease strain on the knees and hands. This position opens the pelvis and uses gravity to help move baby down.

NOTE: Always speak to your health-care provider about what birthing position is best for your delivery in order to understand the risks and benefits so that you and your baby are kept safe.

BIRTHING POSITIONS
BABY IS COMING

COMMON BIRTHING POSITIONS CONTINUED

POSITION 5: **SIDE-LYING**

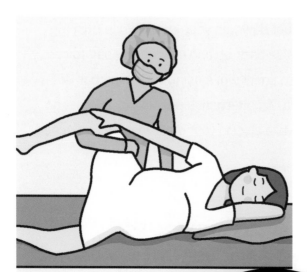

In this position you lie on your side with one of your legs raised, preferably with the help of a midwife, nurse, or your partner. It's simple and easy and allows you to rest while reducing the risk of tearing.

This position can be done with an epidural. However, the position does not utilize gravity well and may result in a longer delivery.

Mommy Hack

Be sure to speak to your doula, midwife, and doctor ahead of delivery to make sure everyone is clear and on the same page as to how you want to deliver.

POSITION 6: **RECLINING**

A common position for delivery, in the reclining position you can rest against a bed, your partner, a birthing ball, or wall. You keep your legs spread wide, knees bent, with feet either flat on the bed or raised in stirrups.

This is a comfortable position for mom-to-be, especially if you have an epidural, but it does not work with gravity and may result in extended delivery times.

There are several reclined positions:

· Lithotomy   · Supine   · Semi-sitting   · Semi-recumbent

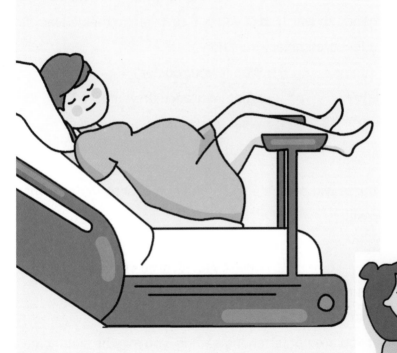

LITHOTOMY POSITION:
Where you are lying flat or somewhat inclined on your back and legs raised, supported in stirrups.

SUPINE POSITION:
When you are lying flat on your back. If in this position your head is somewhat elevated, it may be referred to as **SEMI-SITTING** or **SEMI-RECUMBENT.**

NOTE: Always speak to your health-care provider about what to expect from all delivery options to understand what is right for you and your baby as well as the risks and benefits so that you and your baby are kept safe.

VAGINAL DELIVERY
A BLOW BY BLOW

A step-by-step outline of what typically happens during a normal vaginal delivery.

 NURSES' STATION

One of the first places you will go when you arrive at the hospital is the nurses' station, unless you come into emergency, in which case you will be taken to the delivery floor. A nurse/clerk will ask you a few preliminary questions:

- What are your symptoms?
- What is your due date?
- Do you have any allergies?
- Who is your doctor?
- What insurance do you have?
- What medications do you take?

 TRIAGE

Before you are admitted, a nurse will evaluate your condition to determine in what stage of labor you are. They will:

- Connect a fetal monitor.
- Check your vitals.
- Monitor your contractions.
- Review your health history.
- Check your degree of dilation.

If your water has broken, you may have a speculum exam to confirm.

NOTE: If they determine that you are not far enough along, you may be sent home.

 PAPERWORK

Expect paperwork; you will need to sign multiple forms, even if you preregister.

 LABOR & DELIVERY ROOM

If they determine you are in labor, the doctor will officially admit you as a laboring patient. A nurse will set you up in a labor/delivery room. Blood will be taken, monitors connected, and an IV port put in (in case an IV is needed later). If you have your own gown, you can change into that.

NOTE: Speak to your health-care provider about what to expect from your labor and delivery to understand the process, procedures, and any risks and benefits to determine what is right for you and your baby.

In the room designed for labor, delivery, and postpartum recovery, you will find:

THE BED: Labor and delivery beds are specially made to transform into birthing beds, which can be rolled into the delivery room if you need a C-section.

MEDICAL EQUIPMENT: There are all kinds of medical equipment in your room, very neatly tucked into cabinets to be brought out when needed. A fetal monitor, IV pole, and blood pressure equipment will be next to the bed.

CHAIR: Most rooms have a chair that reclines, which can be used for certain birthing positions and also so that whoever is with you can catch a few Zzzs, if needed.

BATHROOM: The bathroom will have a shower and typically a shower chair. The toilet can be adjusted to collect needed urine samples or turned into a sitz bath to soothe sore private parts.

 SETTLE IN/LABOR

It's time to make yourself comfortable, unpack, and set things up the way you want them for labor. Get your music, find the ice machine, and familiarize yourself with the lighting, nurse call button, bed controls, the vomit bucket, and any other things you think you may need.

As you progress through labor, what happens next depends on your personal pain-management plan.

For a medication-free route, you may walk around, use a birthing ball, take a shower, and utilize a birthing tub to deal with the pain. Nurses will monitor you periodically to check baby's heart rate and your contractions.

QUICK TIP

During your visit to the hospital, ask your guide about the admission process and procedures for their specific facility, parking, drop-off location, rooms, guest policies, etc.

For an epidural route, there's no specific time when it is given; you have to request it. Keep in mind, it's likely to be about 30 to 45 minutes before you actually are pain free.

VAGINAL DELIVERY
A BLOW BY BLOW CONTINUED

QUICK TIP

Uncontrollable shakes during labor and delivery—yes, it's normal. They are thought to be caused by sudden changes in hormones, a drop in body temperature, or an infection.

 SETTLE IN/LABOR

With an epidural, a catheter is inserted in order to empty your bladder.

PROGRESSING THROUGH LABOR

During this time, you will be with your partner and doula (if you are using one) and whoever else is with you. The nursing staff will continue to check in on you, and, of course, if you need any help, you can call them. The labor process is different for everyone, but it may be many hours before you are ready to deliver.

At some point, you will feel some intense pressure, like you have to do number two BADLY! When you do, buzz the nurse to have the OB check on you. You do not want to push until your OB confirms that you are at full dilation (10 cm).

 DELIVERY

If you are ready, things will start speeding up. You will be prepped and your health-care provider will guide you when to push. It might take three to four pushes or twenty to thirty; every delivery is different, but your baby is born! **NOTE:** At this point, your baby's nose and mouth may be suctioned to clear them.

 CORD CLAMPING/CUTTING

Once your baby is born, the umbilical cord is clamped near the belly button and a little farther up the cord and then cut. You can have your partner cut the cord if you like.

DELAYED CLAMPING:

You can choose to delay clamping for 30 seconds to a minute to allow the blood supply from the placenta to flow to the baby before it is cut.

APGAR TEST

Between one and five minutes after birth, this test is done to evaluate your baby's condition: **A**ppearance (skin color), **P**ulse, **G**rimace response (reflexes), **A**ctivity (muscle tone), and **R**espiration.

 SKIN TO SKIN

If your baby is healthy and you want skin-to-skin contact, your doctor will lay the baby on your bare chest right after delivery. Baby can stay there for most of the post-delivery routines.

 STANDARD PROCESSES

Next comes recording your baby's weight, head circumference, and body length. The nurse will take a hand- and footprint and give the baby a bath unless you choose delayed bathing.

DELAYED BATHING:
The World Health Organization recommends delaying bathing for 24 hours. Babies are born covered in a natural white substance called vernix, which has antibacterial and healing properties.

Baby will receive a Vitamin K injection, and antibiotic ointment is placed in the eyes.

 DELIVERING THE PLACENTA

During this time, the doctor will address any tearing if needed while you await the placenta to be delivered.

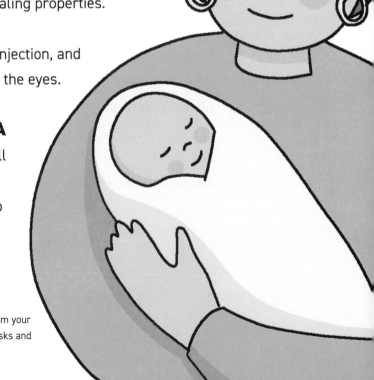

NOTE: Speak to your health-care provider about what to expect from your labor and delivery to understand the process, procedures, and any risks and benefits to determine what is right for you and your baby.

CESAREAN SECTION
WHAT TO KNOW

WHAT IS IT?

CESAREAN SECTION OR C-SECTION: A surgical procedure for delivering a baby. It's done by making an incision/cut in your abdomen and uterus. It is typically done when a vaginal delivery is not possible or safe, or when the health of the mother or the baby is at risk.

ELECTIVE C-SECTION: Occurs when the woman requests a C-section even though there is no medical need for it.

REASONS FOR C-SECTIONS

- High-risk pregnancy.
- Have had a prior C-section.
- A problem with the placenta.
- Baby is breech.
- Baby is too big.
- Expecting multiples.
- Vaginal delivery is too risky.
- Baby has a birth defect.
- Irregular fetal heartbeat.
- Mother has diabetes or HIV.

RISKS OF C-SECTIONS

- Bleeding
- Infection
- Bladder or bowel injury
- Adverse reaction to medicines
- Blood clots
- Future issue with placenta

NOTE: After a C-section, you may not be able to have a vaginal birth for future pregnancies depending on the type of C-section performed. Midline/vertical incisions ON THE UTERUS (not the skin) are not strong enough to withstand labor contractions, making a repeat C-section necessary. The incision on the skin may not match the incision on the uterus, so make sure you are informed about the type of C-section that was performed.

TYPES OF C-SECTIONS

There are two types of C-sections:

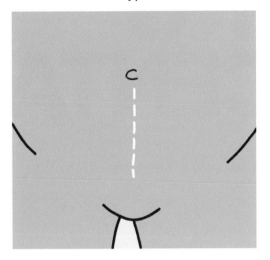

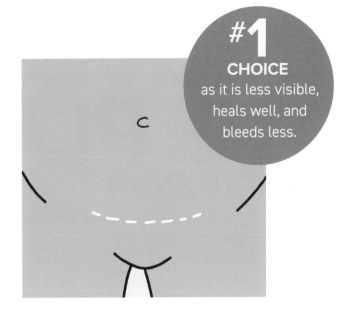

#1 CHOICE as it is less visible, heals well, and bleeds less.

MIDLINE CUT:
This is an up-and-down cut from the belly button to the pubic hairline.

BIKINI CUT:
This is a horizontal cut across the pubic hairline.

C-SECTION PROCEDURE | STEP BY STEP

1. A urinary catheter will be put in, and an IV line will be started in your arm.

2. A strap will be placed over your legs for safety.

3. The hair in the surgical area will be shaved and skin cleaned.

4. A drape is placed over the abdomen to protect the sterile environment.

5. Your vitals will be continuously monitored.

6. Once the anesthesia has taken effect, an incision is made and bleeding sealed.

7. A second, deeper incision is done to reach the uterus, which is then opened.

8. The amniotic sac is opened, and the baby is delivered.

9. The umbilical cord is cut.

10. Medicine is given to help your uterus expel the placenta.

11. The placenta is removed, and the uterus and placenta examined.

12. The incisions in the uterus, then muscle, and finally skin are closed.

13. Bandage is applied.

14. You are moved to a recovery room and monitored until you go back to your room.

Procedure takes **45 min.** Emergency **15–20 min.**

DELIVERING THE PLACENTA

WHAT TO KNOW

Delivering the placenta (also called afterbirth) is also known as the third stage of labor and happens after your baby is born.

WHAT IS IT?

THE PLACENTA: The organ that joins mother and her baby during pregnancy. Oxygen and nutrients pass through it to baby, while waste and carbon monoxide pass through it to the mother.

PLACENTA DELIVERY PERIOD

While awaiting your placenta to be delivered, you and your baby may start to bond, via skin-to-skin contact or possibly your first breastfeeding opportunity.

PLACENTA DELIVERY

Your vagina continues to contract after your baby is born in order to expel the placenta. Most placenta deliveries occur spontaneously within a few minutes of birth, but it can take longer.

In addition to spontaneous delivery, there are two methods, which can be used separately or combined, to help deliver the placenta.

1. ACTIVE MANAGEMENT: A drug is injected soon after your baby is born, which speeds up the delivery of the placenta by stimulating the womb to contract. It also helps prevent bleeding.

NOTE: The information provided is not a substitute for professional medical advice, diagnosis, or treatment. Always consult your obstetrician or primary health-care provider to ensure that a treatment or medication is right and safe for you and your baby.

2. PHYSIOLOGICAL MANAGEMENT: The method most often used by midwives for home births, helping expel the placenta by manually pushing, utilizing gravity, contractions, or nipple stimulation.

If it takes longer than 30 minutes to deliver the placenta, or you are bleeding, a doctor will remove it manually.

DOES DELIVERING THE PLACENTA HURT?

You will experience mild contractions during the delivery process, but they usually don't hurt. Some women don't even realize it's happening; others may experience a slight gush of blood after their baby is delivered, followed by the placenta.

THE FINAL STEPS

1. Once the placenta is out, the doctor or midwife will examine you for tears, if any, and will stitch and clean them. You will likely be given an ice pack to reduce swelling of the perineum.

2. The nurse will help you put on a maxi pad or put some thick pads under your bottom, because you'll still be bleeding. Once you're up for it, you'll be transferred to a postpartum room.

3. Once the placenta is delivered, the health-care professional will examine it to ensure it is intact. It might be sent to pathology for further examination.

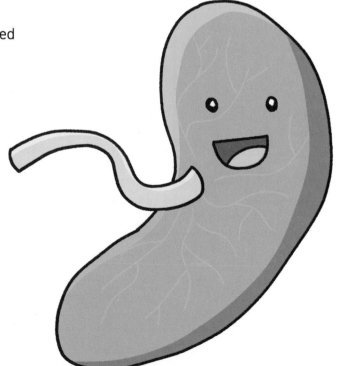

THIS PACKAGE IS OVERDUE

WHEN BABY IS LATE

You have everything ready, the nursery is done, the changing station stocked with diapers, and all the baby gear is standing by—but where is baby?

WHAT IS IT?

A baby is considered late or post-term if it hasn't arrived by week 41 or 42.

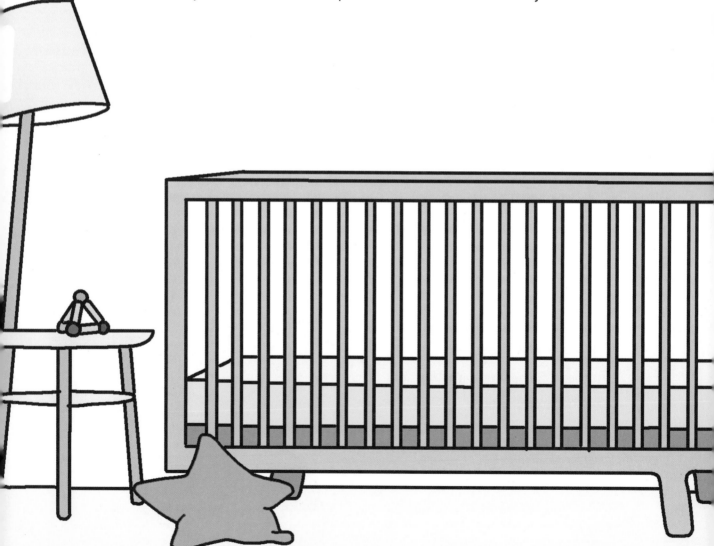

WHAT CAUSES IT?

No one knows why some babies want to hang out a bit longer than others; however, some factors that might result in a late delivery are:

- It is your first pregnancy.
- Your previous babies were born late.
- Family history of late deliveries.

- You're delivering a boy.
- You are overweight.
- Miscalculated due date.

WHAT HAPPENS?

Your doctor continues to monitor you and checks your baby's:

- Size
- Heart rate
- Position
- Movement

WHY INDUCE LABOR?

Your doctor may decide to induce labor after you are one to two weeks past your due date. Doctors do not want you to go too far past your due date, as the risk of health issues starts to go up.

WHAT ARE THE RISKS?

- Need for operative vaginal delivery or C-section.

- Post-maturity syndrome: a decrease in fat under the skin, lack of vernix coating.

- Low amniotic fluid, which can affect heart rate and umbilical cord compression.

- Meconium (baby's first poop) in the baby's lungs.

- Severe vaginal tears.
- Infection.

- Stillbirth risk increases.
- Postpartum bleeding.

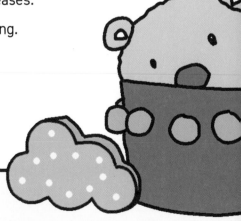

PREMATURE BIRTH

WHAT TO KNOW

Having a premature baby can be very stressful and tough on the parents. Thanks to today's medical advances, many premature babies develop into healthy children who don't even realize they had a tough start in life.

QUICK TIP

A premature baby will need special care when you get home.

Consult with the NICU team and your pediatrician before you leave the hospital.

WHAT IS IT?

PREMATURE BABY: Also called preterm or preemie, a baby that is born too early, before 37 weeks of pregnancy.

MODERATE to LATE PRETERM = 32 TO 37 WEEKS

VERY PRETERM = 28 TO 32 WEEKS

EXTREMELY PRETERM = BEFORE 28 WEEKS

WHAT HAPPENS WHEN PREMATURE?

Premature babies need special medical monitoring and care in a NICU (neonatal intensive care unit).

NOTE:
Depending on how premature your baby is, it may require an infant car bed instead of a car seat.

HEALTH CONCERNS

Premature babies can have many health issues primarily because its organs did not have enough time to develop. The earlier a baby is born, the greater the risk of serious health concerns.

TYPES OF HEALTH ISSUES

Health concerns range from:

- Difficulty breathing
- Intestinal problems
- Temperature control problems
- Cerebral palsy
- Hearing problems
- Heart problems

- Brain hemorrhages
- Learning disabilities
- Feeding difficulties
- Vision problems
- Liver problems
- Blood infections

CAUSES OF PREMATURE BIRTHS

- Chronic health conditions, like diabetes
- Drug or alcohol abuse
- Having multiples, twins, triplets, etc.
- Preeclampsia (high blood pressure)
- Uterine or cervical problems
- Not enough time between pregnancies
- Moms under 20 or over 40 years of age
- Vaginal bleeding or infection
- Smoking while pregnant
- Family history of premature births
- High stress
- Having multiples

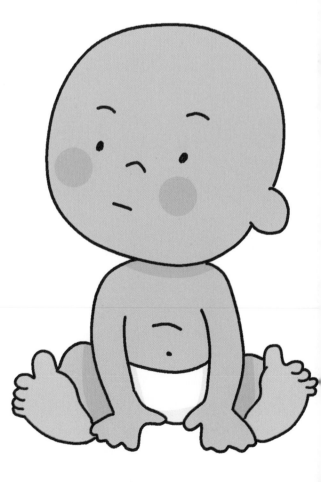

Welcome
to the world
little one.

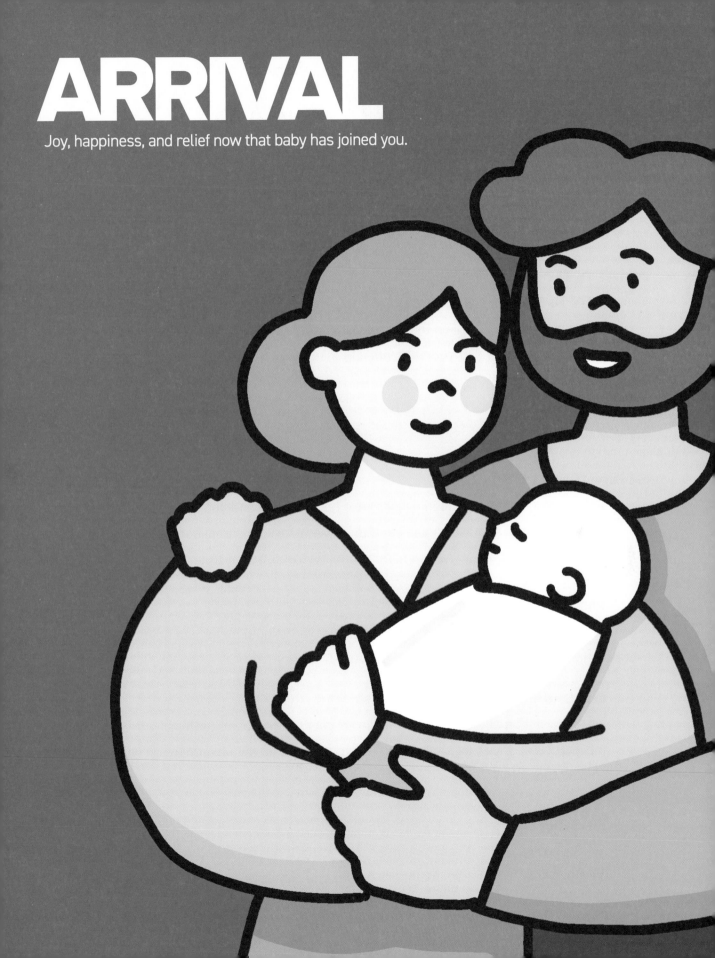

ARRIVAL

Joy, happiness, and relief now that baby has joined you.

SKIN TO SKIN
KANGAROO CARE

Childbirth is a dramatic process for Mom and baby, and skin-to-skin contact has been shown to make the transition smoother for baby.

WHAT IS IT?

SKIN TO SKIN/KANGAROO CARE: Simply means placing the naked or mostly naked baby belly down on the mother's or father's bare chest—you are skin to skin. Cover baby and yourself with a blanket to keep you both warm.

WHO DOES IT?

Both mothers and/or fathers can practice skin-to-skin contact.

WHEN TO DO IT?

Skin-to-skin contact can begin right after baby is born and you are still in the delivery room if you had a full-term baby and there were/are no complications. It is recommended that you have an hour of uninterrupted skin-to-skin time.

VAGINAL DELIVERY:

For a vaginal delivery with no complications, you should be able to have skin-to-skin contact very quickly after baby is delivered.

C-SECTION:

You may still be able to do skin-to-skin contact upon delivery unless your baby needs medical care. Once that's taken care of, you should be able to cuddle up with your baby shortly thereafter.

PRETERM BABY:

Skin-to-skin contact is recommended, but you will need the approval of your health-care provider/NICU team members before you can have skin-to-skin time.

BENEFITS OF SKIN TO SKIN

BONDING

Promotes a stronger connection between Mom, Dad, and baby.

CALMING

Soothes you and your baby; the result is less crying.

WEIGHT GAIN

Has a positive effect on baby's weight gain.

STABILIZING

Releases hormones that reduce stress and stabilizes the baby's body temperature, breathing rate, heart rate, and blood-sugar levels.

HORMONES

Releases mother's hormones, which reduces stress and promotes healing.

BREASTFEEDING

Encourages the production and flow of mom's first milk (colostrum) and leads to more successful breastfeeding.

IMMUNE SYSTEM

Strengthens your baby's immune system.

POSTPARTUM

Lowers the chance and effects of postpartum depression.

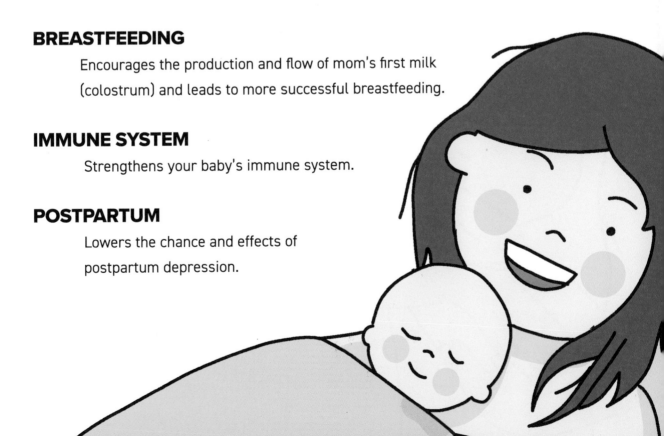

TIME TO EAT
BREASTFEEDING

Thinking about breastfeeding your baby? Here are some things to consider.

QUICK TIP

While touring the hospital, ask about lactation support after delivery and postpartum, helping you perfect your latch. It can make all the difference later!

OVERVIEW

Breastfeeding is a wonderful thing to do, and it has many benefits for both baby and Mom, but NOT every mom is comfortable or successful doing it. It is important to understand that whether you choose to breastfeed or not and for how long you choose to breastfeed are personal choices. Whatever you decide, you should never feel guilty about your decision.

For those of you choosing to breastfeed, it's also important to understand that breastfeeding doesn't come naturally to most women; you will need to learn how to do it, and mastering it can take some practice.

BREASTFEEDING

Breastfeeding, also referred to as nursing, is the process of feeding babies with milk from the mammary glands (a woman's breasts). The baby feeds directly on the breast or from a bottle with milk expressed from the breast using a pump.

ANTENATAL EXPRESSING

A technique of expressing colostrum before the birth of your baby, usually in the final weeks of pregnancy. It can help establish milk production and allow you to have colostrum on hand in case of feeding difficulties in the first days of life (speak to your health-care provider).

WHEN AND FOR HOW LONG?

You can start at any time, but it's recommended that you begin nursing, if you can, within the first hour of your baby's birth. The American Academy of Pediatrics (AAP) recommends that mothers continue breastfeeding exclusively for at least six months, and, if possible, continue breastfeeding along with other food for up to two years or longer.

BENEFITS OF BREASTFEEDING

BONDING:

Nursing can be a special moment between you and your baby.

COLOSTRUM:

This is the first form of breast milk that the mammary glands release. Breast milk is an amazing food for babies because it is super dense with nutrients and high in antibodies and antioxidants to build baby's new immune system. It is thicker and more yellow than regular breast milk, which typically begins to appear two to four days after giving birth.

Health experts and the AAP recommend breastfeeding all infants because of its many health benefits for baby and mother.

Health Benefits for Baby:

- Easily digestible.
- Full of antibodies.
- Highly nutritious.
- Helps prevent diabetes.
- Helps fight infections.
- Reduces risk of obesity.
- Helps prevent diarrhea.
- Fights respiratory infections.
- Reduces risk of asthma.
- Helps prevent childhood cancers.

Health Benefits for Mom

- Reduces the risk of ovarian cancer.
- Reduces risk of postpartum depression.
- Lowers risk of breast cancer.
- Lowers osteoporosis risk.
- Burns calories.

Mommy Hack

Reminder: Your milk may not come in right away—don't be surprised or feel guilty about it. Breastfeeding can be hard!

BREASTFEEDING HOW TO

For the essential steps, practical techniques, and helpful tips on breastfeeding, refer to: *The Simplest Baby Book in the World*

TESTS & SCREENINGS

There are several tests on your newborn done while you are in the hospital. They are routine and help health professionals identify and treat specific conditions that might arise.

SCREENING REQUIREMENTS

All states require certain screenings of newborns. Any decision to decline them should first be discussed with your pediatrician, since newborn screenings are designed to protect the health of your baby.

Even babies who are not born in a hospital need to have newborn screenings performed. If you plan a home birth, the licensed midwife may be qualified to complete the newborn blood test and hearing screening; if not, you will need to have your pediatrician arrange it.

PREEMIE BABY SCREENINGS

Babies born premature, with health conditions or with a low birth weight, often have certain medical problems that require special treatments. These treatments can affect the screening results, requiring a special process and more than one blood draw throughout baby's hospital stay.

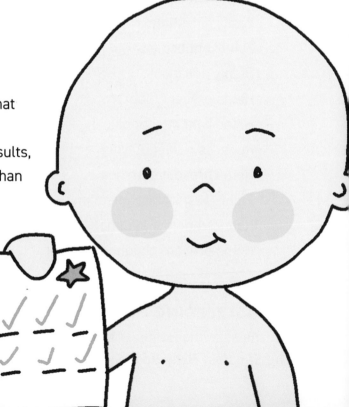

BLOOD TEST HEEL STICK

The heel of the newborn is pricked, and drops of blood are placed on a filter paper, which is sent to the lab.

Here are some disorders that are screened for:
- Phenylketonuria (PKU)
- Cystic fibrosis
- Congenital hypothyroidism
- Maple syrup urine disease
- Sickle cell disease
- Galactosemia
- Homocystinuria
- Congenital Adrenal Hyperplasia

HEARING SCREEN

Two tests can be used to screen for hearing loss in babies:

1. Otacoustic Emission Test
Determines how the baby's ears respond to sound. A small earpiece or probe is placed in the baby's ear, and sounds are played. When hearing is normal, sound waves travel back through the ear canal. These are measured by the earpiece. If no echo is detected, that can indicate potential hearing loss.

2. Auditory Brain Stem Response
This test evaluates the brain's response to sound. During this test, miniature earphones are placed in the baby's ears, and sounds are played. Electrodes placed on baby's scalp track and measure the brain's response to those sounds, determining if there is any hearing loss.

PULSE OXIMETRY TEST

Measures how much oxygen is in the blood.

Sensors are placed on the baby's hand or foot to measure the heart rate and blood oxygen level.

Low blood oxygen levels can identify babies who may have Critical Congenital Heart Disease (CCHD). The test is painless and takes a few minutes; typically done when the baby is at least 24 hours of age.

QUICK TIP

With a home birth, some of these tests may be done at your two-day checkup with the midwife or doctor.

MULTIPLES
TWINS AND MORE

Being pregnant with multiples means you will need to take special care of yourself.

Mommy Hack

NOTE: Your birthing expectation may get turned upside down because even if one baby delivers normally, the second could flip breech and may require a C-section.

WHAT IS IT?

MULTIPLE PREGNANCY: When you are pregnant with more than one baby at a time.

TYPES

TWINS: Carrying two babies.

IDENTICAL TWINS: When a single egg is fertilized by one sperm that divides into two zygotes.

FRATERNAL TWINS: When two eggs are fertilized by two sperm.

TRIPLETS: Carrying three babies.

QUADRUPLETS: Carrying four babies.

QUINTUPLETS: Carrying five babies.

HOW IT HAPPENS

There are two main ways that a multiple pregnancy happens.

· One egg splits before it implants in the uterus.

· Two or more separate eggs are fertilized by different sperm at the same time.

INCREASED CHANCES OF MULTIPLES IF:

· You are over 30 years of age.

· You are a twin yourself or have twins in your family.

· You are using fertility drugs.

COMPLICATIONS

- Increased risk of premature labor
- Increased risk of premature birth
- Gestational diabetes
- Low baby birth weight
- Anemia
- Liver issues
- Increased risk of stillbirth

- Preeclampsia
- Gestational high blood pressure
- Placenta abruption
- Increased likelihood of C-section
- More severe morning sickness
- Increased risk of miscarriage
- Increased heartburn

THINGS TO DO

If you are carrying multiples, you should be sure to:

- Get enough liquids.
- Get plenty of rest and sleep.
- Get good prenatal care.
- Take prescribed vitamins.

- Eat healthy, nutritious foods.
- Eat plenty of protein.
- Do low-impact exercise.

QUICK TIP
EATING FOR TWO
If you are pregnant with twins, you will need about 600 extra calories a day—that is 300 calories for each baby.

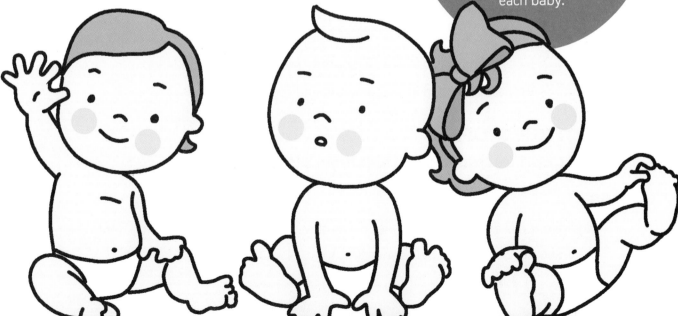

AND THIS BABY MAKES TWO
HAVING YOUR SECOND BABY

Here are some things you need to know the second time around.

Mommy Hack

Help the transition by reading books to your toddler about having a sibling. Give a gift to the sibling from the newborn after it is is born.

THINGS TO KNOW

IT WON'T BE LIKE THE FIRST

No two pregnancies are the same. This time around things may be different. You may have had horrible morning sickness during your first, but with the second, it may well be much easier.

LABOR WILL BE FASTER

Many times, labor and delivery are easier and faster with the second baby.

PREPARE BABY ONE FOR BABY TWO

There will be things that you will need to lay the groundwork for:

- If firstborn is two to three years old, consider transiting out of crib.
- Reading books on the arrival of a new baby to your toddler can help prepare them.
- If firstborn is around 18–24 months, train or lay the foundation of potty training.
- Prepare first born for baby noises and crying.

YOU GOT THE STUFF

Good news! You are not going to have to buy all the stuff you did with the first one.

GUILT

You might feel a bit guilty about not being able to give the same amount of attention to your second child as you did to your first.

AFTER LABOR PAIN

You may experience stronger after-labor pain with your second baby.

SIBLING JEALOUSY

Your firstborn may wonder why they are not getting your undivided attention and will try very hard to get it back. The firstborn may also try acting a bit like a baby in an attempt to get your attention.

EXHAUSTING

Being super honest—you thought you were tired with baby number one, well, sorry to say, now with two, it's going be really tough. All the exhaustion you had with baby one, now you have that and another child to look after.

OUT AND ABOUT

This also gets more complicated. Keeping an eye on both kids at the same time while at the park or shopping is hard.

PERFECT PARENT

Now that you have baby number two, you will find that some things—well—you just let them slide a bit. All that stress about having and doing it perfectly the first time is just much less important the second time.

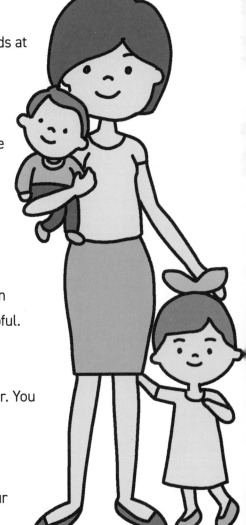

SUPPORT

With baby number two, you will need all the support you can get. Your friends and family (your village) can be really helpful.

YOU'RE SHOWING

Typically, with your second baby, you will be showing sooner. You also may be carrying lower this time around.

IT'S A PAIN

Unfortunately, your aches and pains might be worse, as your muscles are looser, resulting in more back and pelvic pain.

EATING THE PLACENTA
WHAT TO CONSIDER AND KNOW

What to know about placentophagy.

WHAT IS IT?

PLACENTOPHAGY: The eating of part or all of the placenta after giving birth.

HOW?

There are several ways one could consume the placenta.

- **ENCAPSULATION**

    The placenta is dehydrated, ground up, and put in capsules (pill).

- **EATING IT RAW**

    Sometimes put in a smoothie.

- **EATING IT COOKED**

    There are various recipes for preparing placenta online.

WHY?

People who recommend it believe that it has health benefits; however, at this time, there is little research and data to support the benefits claimed.

BELIEVED BENEFITS:

- Increased milk production
- Improved postnatal mood
- Preventing anemia
- Increased energy
- Helps manage after-birth pain

NOTE: Always speak to your health-care provider/professional about the risk involved and what is safe and right for you and your pregnancy.

WARNING:

The Centers for Disease Control and Prevention (CDC) warns against consuming the placenta because the baby could develop Group B streptococcus, thought to be the result of the mother consuming contaminated placenta capsules. There is also concern that no standardized process for preparing and/or improper handling of the placenta can potentially lead to illness. Group B streptococcus can be a life-threatening infection for infants.

Because of the risk of infection, some hospitals do not allow you to consume or take the placenta. Check with your hospital ahead of time to understand their policies regarding it.

NOTE: Speak with your health-care provider if you are considering placentophagy to understand if it is safe for you and baby.

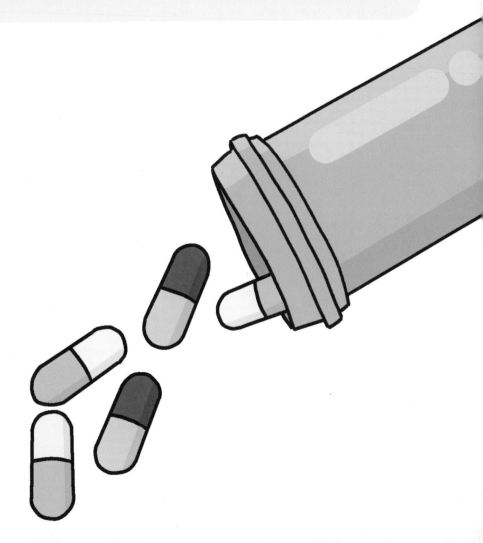

Taking care
of you is taking
care of your
family.

RECOVERY

The postpartum period for Mom and baby.

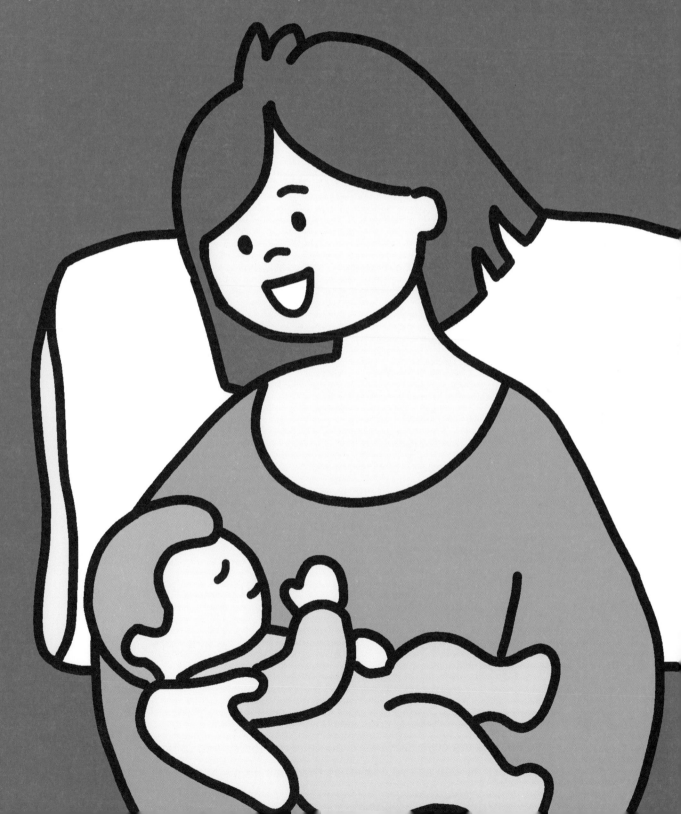

RECOVERY
TIME TO HEAL

You have just done one of the most AMAZING things: brought a new life into the world. It's taken a lot out of you physically and emotionally, and now it is time to heal. Like your pregnancy, your postpartum recovery will be unique to you.

WHAT IS IT?

POSTPARTUM: Literally means following childbirth.

The postpartum period begins immediately after childbirth. Each person's postpartum is different and depends on the individual, the type of delivery—vaginal or C-section—and if there were any complications.

POSTPARTUM RECOVERY

Now that you have welcomed the newest member of your family, you will face a whole new set of challenges:

- Caring for your tiny newborn
- Caring for YOURSELF
- Hormonal changes (again)
- Lack of sleep
- Breastfeeding (if you choose to)

Keep in mind that healing is a process that takes time; be patient and gentle with yourself.

The postpartum period typically lasts from delivery up to 8 to 12 weeks, but the time frame is unique to you.

POSTPARTUM ADVICE

In this section, we cover the major postpartum topics and things you need to know and consider as well as provide ideas that may help you heal.

Taking care
of
yourself
doesn't mean
me first;
it means
me too.

THE MUST-HAVES
POSTPARTUM RECOVERY

Practical suggestions for common postpartum issues.

Mommy Hack

KEEP RECEIPTS

You may not have a vaginal delivery, as expected, but a C-section—in which case, some of the items you purchased might need to be returned.

GET THE RIGHT STUFF!

Scan the QR code to easily get our recommendations for everything you will need to recover.

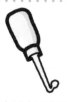

PERI BOTTLE

This bottle is used to clean your vaginal and rectal areas after delivery. It is designed to gently squirt water on your private parts.

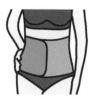

BELLY WRAP

These garments are intended to help recovery after a C-section. They support the muscles and organs. Look for a fitted, waterproof cover that is breathable and hypoallergenic. Consult your doctor to see if it is right for you.

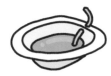

SITZ BATH

For tearing or an episiotomy, you may want to take sitz baths to ease pain and itching as well as reduce swelling and ease hemorrhoids. You can take a sitz bath in the bathtub or purchase a version that sits over the toilet.

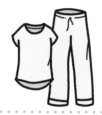

COMFY PAJAMAS

Having PJs or lounge wear that provide the utmost comfort is a must while pregnant. Best are ones that are lightweight made from organic silk, soft flannel, or cotton.

STOOL SOFTENER

After delivery, passing those first poos can be really difficult and painful. A stool softener is a medication that softens your bowel movement by adding more moisture to it, making it easier to pass.

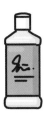

WITCH HAZEL/WITCH HAZEL PADS

Witch hazel will help reduce the swelling, pain, and bruising in your vaginal area.

PAIN-RELIEVING SPRAY | NUMBING AGENT

Soothing/numbing agents come in the form of a spray, cream, or ointment and are used to ease the pain and itching of the vaginal region postpartum.

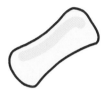

MAXI PADS

You will want a pad that is super absorbent, extra wide, and long. There are scented and unscented versions depending on what you like.

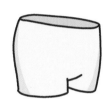

POSTPARTUM UNDERWEAR

Bleeding in the days and weeks after delivery is heavy, and you will likely ruin a pair or two of underwear—better to have ones you can throw away. Some models have a pocket for an ice pack.

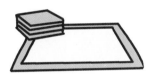

PEE PADS

Consider getting the absorbent pads used for absorbing dog accidents. You can use them over your sheet and mattress so that, if you leak, you won't ruin your sheets.

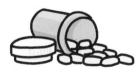

PAIN MEDICINE

You will want to have pain medication available; ibuprofen is recommended by the ACOG, because little of it passes through to your breast milk. Talk to your OB-GYN about your options for pain relief before leaving the hospital.

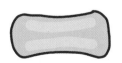

COOLING PADS

Essentially a sanitary napkin that has been chilled in the freezer, which you can place in your underwear to relieve pain. They also come premade.

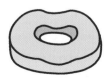

DONUT PILLOW

If you had any vaginal lacerations or hemorrhoids, you are going to want one of these to sit on while you heal.

POSTPARTUM CHECKUP

WHAT TO EXPECT

Whether vaginal or C-section delivery, you will experience postpartum bleeding and discharge. It's normal but stressful. Here is what you need to know and do during this time.

WHAT IS IT?

A POSTPARTUM CHECKUP: A medical checkup a new mom gets after having a baby to make sure her recovery is going well—physically and mentally.

WHY?

This checkup is very important because new moms are at risk for many serious and sometimes life-threatening health complications.

It is especially important for mothers-to-be who have experienced a loss, a miscarriage, stillbirth, or a neonatal death. Your doctor might also connect you with a genetic counselor or mental health provider to determine if there is some underlying cause that could affect another pregnancy.

WHEN?

Typically, this appointment is scheduled for six weeks after your delivery, although the American College of Obstetricians & Gynecologists recommends that you see your OB-GYN or midwife sooner, around three weeks after delivery.

BRINGING ALONG BABY?

You usually can bring your baby along to these appointments, but it is best to confirm this with your health-care provider. If you do bring your baby, you should arrange your appointment for a time when your newborn is not overly tired or hungry.

WHAT HAPPENS AT THIS APPT.

PELVIC EXAM

Just as you have an annual physical, you will have a pelvic exam to check your vagina (birth canal), uterus, and cervix, and at the same time, you should have a pap smear.

BREAST EXAM

This is very important because new moms are at risk for many serious and sometimes life-threatening health complications.

CHECKING VITALS

You will have a series of standard tests, including weight and blood pressure.

NUTRITIONAL QUESTIONS

Your health-care provider will check your diet to see if you need a supplement like calcium or iron—especially if you are breastfeeding.

HEALTH CONDITIONS

If you had any conditions—for example, gestational diabetes, high blood pressure, or a thyroid condition—your doctor will examine you and may do tests for these conditions.

EPISIOTOMY OR C-SECTION CHECK

If you had one of these procedures, your health-care provider will examine you to ensure you are healing properly.

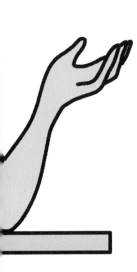

BONDING & THE BLUES

Your practitioner will talk with you to see how you are adapting to having a new baby and how well you are bonding with it. They will look for signs of depression.

SEX TALK

It's a good time to talk about having sex again and using birth control.

QUESTIONS

Be prepared with questions you have.

LOCHIA
POSTPARTUM BLEEDING & CLOTS

Whether you had a vaginal or C-section delivery, you will experience postpartum bleeding and discharge. It is normal, but it is stressful. Here is what you need to know and do during this time.

LOCHIA, VAGINAL DELIVERY (Lasts 4–6 weeks)

Lochia is the name given to the vaginal discharge that occurs after childbirth. This discharge is the result of the body clearing out and restoring the uterus. It's a combination of blood, uterine tissue, amniotic fluid, mucus, and white blood cells. Lochia is mostly blood at first, but as the days pass, it steadily becomes mostly mucus.

3 STAGES OF LOCHIA

STAGE 1: **Lochia Rubra** (Begins day 1–3)

- Bright or dark-red blood.
- Bleeding is heaviest during this stage.
- Mild cramping or contractions as uterus returns to its original size.
- Blood clots ranging in size (from a grape to a golf ball).
- Smells like that of normal menstrual blood.
- Lasts three to four days.

STAGE 2: **Lochia Serosa** (Begins day 4–10)

- Blood/discharge is pinkish or brownish in color.
- Clots smaller than Stage 1 or may disappear completely.
- Bleeding should decrease.
- Lasts 4 to 12 days.

STAGE 3: **Lochia Alba** (Begins day 11–14)

- Discharge is whitish yellow in color.
- May be some spotting of blood.
- Cramping/contractions should be easing off.
- Lasts about 12 days to 6 weeks.

Mommy Hack
TAKE IT SLOW!
You may begin to have light bleeding and think, I'm good to go, can start doing more activities, and then suddenly start having heavy bleeding again.

NOTE: The information provided is not a substitute for professional medical advice, diagnosis, or treatment. Always consult your obstetrician or primary health-care provider to ensure that a treatment or medication is right and safe for you and your baby.

LOCHIA, C-SECTION DELIVERY

After a Cesarean delivery, you will have less lochia than if you had a vaginal delivery, but for a few weeks you will still have some bloody discharge. Over that time, it will go from red to brown to yellow, and finally, to clear, just as a vaginal delivery does.

BLEEDING: What to do?

QUICK TIP

Before leaving the hospital, you will be offered several things for your recovery. Take whatever the hospital offers. You can even ask for extras.

1. In the beginning, bleeding will probably be heavy enough that you'll want to wear a heavy-duty pad or the adult diapers the hospital provides.

2. As the bleeding slows, you can transition to a regular menstrual pad.

3. Change pads often to prevent infection.

4. No tampons: do not use a tampon until your doctor tells you it is OK.

5. Once the discharge is clear and light, you can use a panty liner.

BLEEDING: Why is it increasing?

• **BREASTFEEDING:** Nursing produces hormones which stimulate contractions that can increase bleeding.

• **EXERCISE:** Physical activity, walking, or climbing stairs.

• **STRAINING:** Peeing or pooing can cause bleeding.

• **GETTING UP:** After lying down or sitting, you can have a little bleeding when getting up.

CALL THE DOCTOR

· If you experience heavy bleeding that soaks through a hospital heavy-duty pad/diaper in an hour and doesn't slow.

· If you experience bright red bleeding beyond day three.

· Large-size blood clots bigger than a golf ball, or passing large clots after 24 hours.

· If you experience weakness, dizziness, or feeling faint.

· If you experience blurred vision or rapid heartbeat.

· If you experience bad-smelling or greenish lochia.

POSTPARTUM HAIR LOSS
SHEDDING SOME LIGHT ON IT

Unfortunately, hair loss after pregnancy is common. Learn why it happens and how to treat it.

QUICK TIP

Be gentle with your hair, especially while brushing and washing it. If you don't have one, get a detangling brush that won't pull your hair.

WHAT'S HAPPENING?

A few months after welcoming your little bundle of joy, you notice your hair starts shedding at an alarming rate. YIKES!

Postpartum hair loss is usually an unwelcome surprise for most new moms.

WHY?

Hair tends to grow in cycles—transitioning from a growing cycle, to resting cycle, to shedding cycle. During pregnancy, your hair is in a continuous growth phase (even in all the places you don't want hair to grow)—all due to hormones.

Once those hormones return to normal, all that extra hair begins a shedding phase. Because so much hair is shedding at once, it seems as if it's all coming out, but rest assured, it is normal and will fill back in, usually in a year (yes, I know, it seems like a long time).

WARNING

With all the hair loss, you want to be on the lookout for potential hair tourniquets.

HAIR TOURNIQUETS: Formed when a strand of hair wraps around a baby's fingers, toes, or other parts of the body, cutting off circulation.

TIPS FOR REGAINING FULL HAIR

USE VOLUMIZING SHAMPOO

These shampoos contain ingredients that coat the hair and make them appear fuller. Consider selective conditioning of only the ends.

NO CONDITIONING SHAMPOOS

This type of product tends to weigh your hair down, making it look flat and limp.

USE CONDITIONER FOR THIN HAIR

Use conditioners formulated for fine hair; they tend to be lighter.

HAIR STYLE

Speak to your stylist about hair styles that look fuller—possibly a shorter cut.

BE GENTLE

Take it easy when washing, brushing, or styling it. Take a break from chemical treatments, perms, or straightening for a while. Also, skip the heat from blow dryers, curling irons, or flat irons.

EAT WELL

Make sure you get the right nutrition; continue taking prenatal vitamins to keep hair healthy.

HAIR ACCESSORIES

Avoid elastic bands—use scrunchies or barrettes—and don't pull your hair too tight.

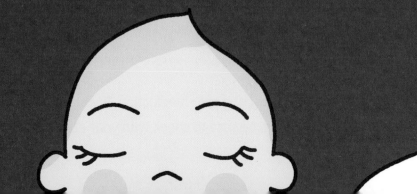

PERINEAL LACERATION

CARING FOR TEARING

Perineal tears happen during childbirth. Here is what you need to know to care for lacerations.

WHAT IS IT?

PERINEAL LACERATION OR VAGINAL TEAR: An injury to the tissue around the vagina and rectum caused by childbirth. This tear is typically closed with stitches that dissolve in five to six weeks; if the tear is small, it may be allowed to heal on its own.

RECOVERY

Until it heals, it can be uncomfortable or painful, depending on the severity of the tear.

Mommy Hack

Create a **PADSICLE:** basically a sanitary napkin that's chilled in the freezer and then placed in your underwear to relieve pain and promote healing.

HEALING TIME IS TYPICALLY
4–6 WEEKS RECOVERY

The amount of time will vary from person to person and on the severity of the tear.

PAIN

Pain and soreness are likely to occur while:

- Sitting
- Urinating
- Walking
- Bowel Movements

TIPS FOR CARING FOR A PERINEAL TEAR

PAIN MEDICATION:

Your doctor likely will prescribe pain medication. If you are taking any other over-the-counter pain medications, be sure to check with your doctor.

STAY HYDRATED:

Drink eight glasses of water each day to avoid constipation and strained bowel movements.

FIBER, FIBER, FIBER:

Eat a diet with lots of fruits and vegetables; you may also take a fiber supplement.

MEDICATIONS:

Be sure to check with your doctor about any regular medication that you take.

ICE IT:

Place a cold pack on the sore area for 10 to 20 minutes at a time. Be sure to put a thin cloth between the ice and your skin.

TAKE A SITZ BATH:

Sitting in three to four inches/1.9 cm of warm water for 15 to 20 minutes, three times a day, will help ease the pain. After bowel movements, pat dry; do not wipe.

AVOID SQUATS:

You will want to avoid putting pressure on the area with any wide leg positions like squats, sitting cross-legged, or going up stairs two at a time. Also, no heavy lifting.

PERI BOTTLE:

Use a peri bottle to clean the area after going to the toilet. Fill the bottle with lukewarm water, and point the stream at the area to wash it while peeing. It will help reduce the stinging sensation.

PADS:

Change your pad often to keep the area clean and dry to protect against infection.

DONUT PILLOW:

Sitting on a pillow can be helpful; some moms use their breastfeeding pillow instead of buying a donut.

SHOWER OR BATHE:

Take a shower or bath every day. You can use a handheld shower head to gently wash the wound, but do not rub soap into the wound.

NOTE: Always speak to your health-care provider about any treatment or medication to understand the risks and benefits so that you and your baby are kept safe.

LETTING THE AIRING OUT
POSTPARTUM GAS

After giving birth, many women experience postpartum gas and bloating. Here is what you can do about it.

POSTPARTUM GAS

It is increased gas and bloating that occurs after having a baby. It can happen whether you have a vaginal or Cesarean delivery, and it typically lasts about a month.

SYMPTOMS

- Flatulence or farting
- Belching
- Sharp abdominal pain
- Abdominal cramps

CAUSES

Experiencing postpartum gas and bloating is a fairly common occurrence, but it also can be related to an underlying health condition that reduces your control over bloating and gas; among them are:

- **PELVIC FLOOR INJURY**

  Pregnancy and delivery stretch and potentially injure the muscles and nerves of the pelvic floor.

- **EPISIOTOMY OR SEVERE PERINEAL LACERATION**

  An episiotomy can weaken the pelvic floor muscles, leading to gas.

- **CONSTIPATION:**

  After childbirth, constipation that can lead to bloating and gas is common.

- **HORMONES**

  The decrease in hormones can slow down digestion, resulting in gas.

- **DIET**

    Eating a diet high in lactose, fructose, sorbitol, or soluble fiber, like dairy products, vegetables, fruits, processed food, and beans can increase gas.

- **HEALTH CONDITIONS**

    Conditions like Crohn's disease, diverticulitis, or ulcerative colitis can result in increased gas.

POSSIBLE REMEDIES

EXERCISE

Moving can help clear things up, but speak to your doctor before beginning any exercise regimen; remember, you are still healing. Try walking and yoga positions, like the cat pose, and pelvic floor exercises.

INCREASED FIBER/LIQUIDS

Constipation contributes to bloating and gassiness, so eating a diet high in non-soluble fiber and staying well-hydrated can help.

MEDICATIONS

An anti-gas medication can help relieve gas pain. However, some pain medications can actually cause constipation. Speak to your doctor about the right medications for you.

BODY POSITIONS

Changing your body position may help you release the gas.

WARM THINGS UP

Warm liquids, herbal teas, or broth may help, as will a warm bath or heating pad.

ABDOMINAL MASSAGE

Try gently massaging your stomach in a clockwise motion.

I'M BACK
MENSTRUATION AFTER DELIVERY

As your body recovers and things start to get back to "normal," you will experience your first period, which is called a postpartum period. Here's what you need to know.

QUICK TIP

Although continuous breastfeeding slows the return of your period and reduces fertility, it's NOT a guarantee that you won't get pregnant.

WHEN

When you get your first period post-delivery depends a lot on if you are breastfeeding, but even that is not a guarantee.

BREASTFEEDING:

If you are breastfeeding continuously, you may not get your period for several months, or until you stop nursing.

BREASTFEEDING PART-TIME:

If you begin breastfeeding part-time—for example, not feeding at night—you may start to get your period.

BOTTLE-FEEDING:

If you bottle feed, you will get your period, possibly as soon as six to eight weeks.

POST-BIRTH BLEEDING

Not all bleeding after delivery is your period. You can expect to have bleeding (lochia) for six to eight weeks after delivery, whether you had a vaginal or Cesarean delivery.

POST-BIRTH PERIOD

Your first periods after the birth of your child may be somewhat different than those you had in the past. You may experience:

- Heavier flow.
- More or less cramping and pain.
- Clotting at first (if it lasts more than a week, see your doctor).
- Irregular cycle length, if you are breastfeeding only periodically.

YOUR PERIOD, YOUR MILK

When your period returns, it will affect your breast milk:

- The milk supply might decrease.
- The taste of your milk may change.

GETTING PREGNANT?

Even though it's not common, it is possible to become pregnant as soon as three weeks after giving birth, even if you are breastfeeding and your period hasn't started yet. That's why it's important that you use some kind of birth control unless you want to get pregnant.

Getting pregnant too soon after childbirth comes with potential risks, such as:

- Premature birth
- Placenta problems
- Low birth weight
- Anemia
- Autism
- Schizophrenia
- Congenital disorders

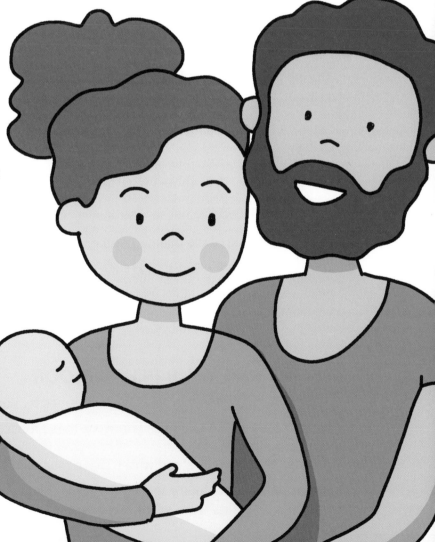

KEGEL EXERCISES
GETTING STARTED

One of the first exercises that you are likely to do are Kegel exercises. Within a few days after a normal vaginal delivery, you may be encouraged to walk or do Kegels.

WHAT IS IT?

KEGEL EXERCISES: These exercises strengthen the muscles of the pelvic floor, which support the uterus, bladder, small intestine, and rectum.

WHY DO THEM?

During pregnancy and childbirth, these muscles are stretched and weakened, which can result in:

- Loss of bladder control and leakage.
- Passing wind from the anus or vagina.
- Failing to reach the toilet in time.
- Reduced vaginal sensation.
- Bulging of the opening of the vagina.
- Repeated urinary tract infections.
- Pain during sex.
- Bowel leakage.

STRENGTHENING YOUR PELVIC FLOOR

You can strengthen your pelvic floor muscles by doing exercises designed specifically to work those muscles.

An easy way to understand where these muscles are: the next time you urinate, try to stop the flow—those are the ones.

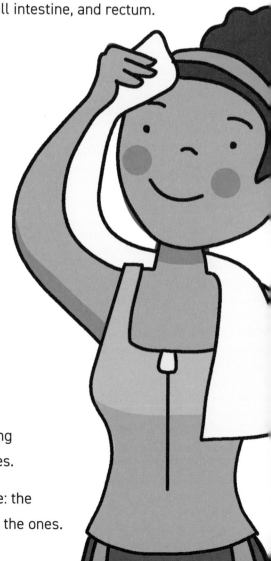

PELVIC FLOOR EXERCISES

STANDARD KEGEL

To strengthen your pelvic floor muscles:

- Sit comfortably and focus on the muscles that stop urination.
- Tighten and squeeze the muscles—it should feel like the muscles are lifting.
- Hold this position for 5 to 10 seconds.
- Release; rest a couple of seconds.
- Repeat 10 to 15 times.

QUICK RELEASE KEGEL

Same as above, but hold for only one second and release. Repeat the exercise ten times, rest, and then begin again. Three sets total.

QUICK TIP

It can take up to six to twelve months to lose your baby fat and get back to your normal weight—so be patient with yourself.

BRIDGE

While strengthening the buttocks, it also helps with the pelvic floor muscles.

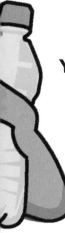

SQUATS

Squatting promotes a stronger pelvic floor, quads, hamstrings, and glutes.

YOGA

Yoga practice can be help strengthen and stabilize the pelvic floor muscles. Certain poses specifically work the pelvic floor muscles:

- Constructive rest pose
- Knees-to-chest pose
- Wide-legged forward fold
- Happy baby pose
- Cat-cow pose
- Warrior II pose
- Wide-legged squat pose

WARNING

Before doing any exercise, consult your health-care provider to make sure a specific exercise is right for your body and recovery.

POSTPARTUM EXERCISES

GETTING PRE-BABY BODY BACK

Exercise can be challenging after delivery—with a new baby to care for, lack of sleep, and the healing process—but it's important and will aid your recovery.

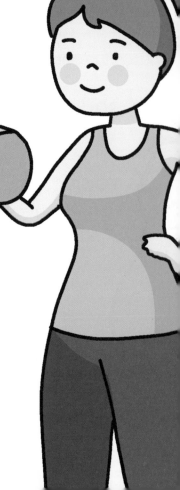

QUICK TIP

Be realistic! No matter how hard core an exercise person you were befor pregnancy, you need to EASE back into it now. Taking the time to rest before you begin is important.

DOCTOR'S OK

Number one: get your doctor's green light before you do any exercise to ensure that you don't do more harm than good.

GENERAL RECOMMENDATION

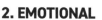

6–8 WEEKS REST

BEFORE BEGINNING EXERCISE

WHY

Postpartum exercises have a wide range of benefits:

1. BODY

- Strengthens muscles.
- Helps lose weight.
- Regains abdominal strength.
- Boosts energy.
- Improves sleep.
- Promotes healing and recovery.

2. EMOTIONAL

- Helps manage stress.
- Improves your mood.
- Reduces depression.

TIPS FOR EXERCISING POSTPARTUM

START SLOWLY:

Ease into an exercise routine, and gradually increase your activity day by day.

CHOOSE THE RIGHT EXERCISE:

Putting too much pressure on your abdomen or perineal area can inhibit or have a negative impact on healing. Consult your health-care provider to determine what are the right exercises for you.

WEAR THE RIGHT CLOTHING:

Look for clothes that provide support but are not too tight.

WAIT TILL THE BLEEDING STOPS:

Before starting an exercise routine, be certain you are no longer bleeding. If you experience bleeding or pain, speak with your health-care provider.

THE WOBBLIES:

You may still have some wobbly joints, so be careful as you exercise.

STAY HYDRATED:

Drink plenty of water; this can't be said enough.

BEGIN WITH LIGHT-TO-MODERATE EXERCISE:

Start with easy-to-do-exercises, like walking. Later, swimming and Pilates are other potentially good exercises, but, as always, check with your health-care provider.

Mommy Hack

If you are breastfeeding, empty your breasts before working out; either nurse or pump.

Wear a support bra for your workouts.

WARNING

Before doing any exercise, check with your health-care provider to make sure any specific exercise is right for your body and your recovery.

EXERCISES
BYE-BYE BELLY

Here is a list of some of the best postpartum exercises after a healthy, uncomplicated vaginal delivery. Always check with your health-care provider to make sure you are ready to start any exercise program.

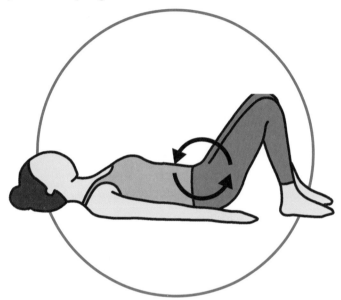

PELVIC TILT

Lie on your back, knees bent, and feet flat on the floor. Tighten your abdominal muscles and roll your hips up toward your head, pressing your back into the floor. Hold for a couple seconds and release.
Repeat 5 to 10 times.

Strengthens: Abdominal muscles and glutes.

DEEP BREATHING ABDOMINAL CONTRACTIONS

Lie on your back with your knees bent and feet flat on the floor. Place one hand on your upper chest and the other under your rib cage. Breathe in slowly through your nose, so your stomach and the hand under your rib cage rise, while the hand on your chest remains still. Tighten your abdominal muscles as you breathe out, causing your hand to fall.
Repeat 10 to 15 times.

Strengthens: Pelvic floor and abdominals.

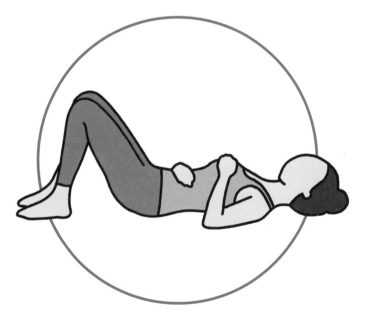

WARNING: Before doing any exercise, consult with your health-care provider to make sure the specific exercise is right for your body and your recovery.

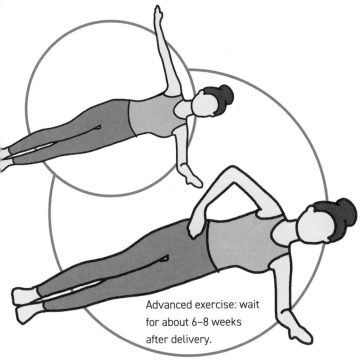

Advanced exercise: wait for about 6–8 weeks after delivery.

SIDE PLANK

Lie on your stomach with your forearm on the floor, elbows under shoulders, and flex feet with toes on the floor. Roll over to one side so that only one forearm is on the floor and you are in a sideways position. Raise your top leg and arm, and hold them in the air for 10 to 20 seconds. Switch sides and repeat with the opposite leg and arm.

Repeat 3 to 4 times.

Strengthens: Glutes, obliques, legs, and shoulders.

PLANK

With your stomach and forearms flat on the floor, and your elbows under your shoulders, raise up on your toes, lifting your hips and stomach off the floor while keeping your back straight, with only your forearms and toes on the floor. Hold for a couple seconds.

Repeat 2 to 3 times.

Strengthens: The core, tightens glutes, and upper body.

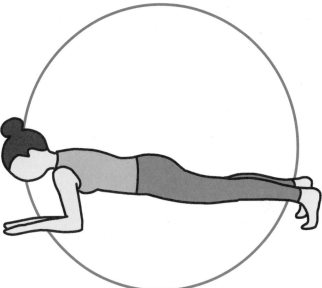

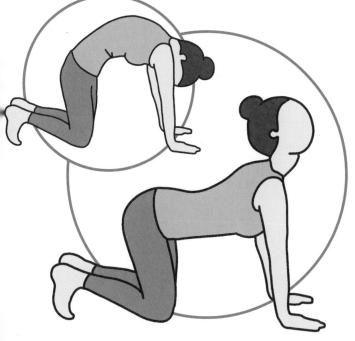

CAT-COW

While on all fours, start with your back flat, head looking down. Keep your hands flat on the floor directly under your shoulders, knees under hips. Take a deep breath in, and, while exhaling, arch your back toward the ceiling, dropping your head. Hold for one to two seconds. Then inhale, lowering your back toward the floor while raising your chin and tailbone toward the ceiling.

Repeat 2 to 3 times.

Strengthens: Back muscles and your core.

EXERCISES

BYE-BYE BELLY CONTINUED

Here is a list of some of the best postpartum exercises after a healthy, uncomplicated vaginal delivery. Always check with your health-care provider to make sure you are ready to start any exercise program.

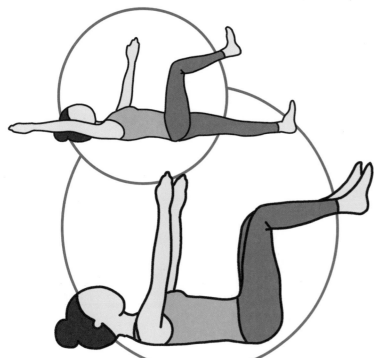

DEAD BUG

Lie flat on your back with your arms held out in front of you, pointing at the ceiling. Bring your legs up so that your knees are bent at 90-degree angles. Slowly lower your right arm and left leg simultaneously, exhaling as you go. Keep going until your arm and leg are just above the floor; be careful not to raise your back off the ground. Slowly return to the starting position and repeat with the opposite arm and leg.

Repeat 10 times.

Strengthens: Abdominals and your core.

SQUATS

Stand with your feet shoulder-width apart. Extend your hands out in front of you. Bend at your knees, your butt should be pointing backward (as if you were going to be sitting on a chair). Knees should be behind your toes. Stand back up. Here's a simpler version: lean back against a wall, feet shoulder-width apart, knees bent at right angles above ankles; hold for 20 seconds. Stand up and rest for 30 seconds.

Repeat 5–7 times.

Strengthens Legs, glutes, quads, hamstrings, and calves; good for the back and abdominal muscles.

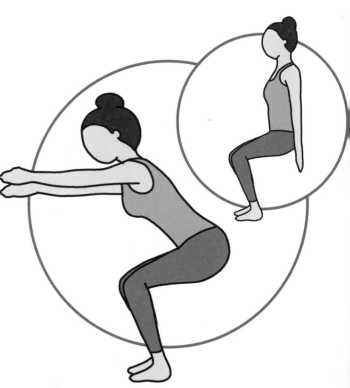

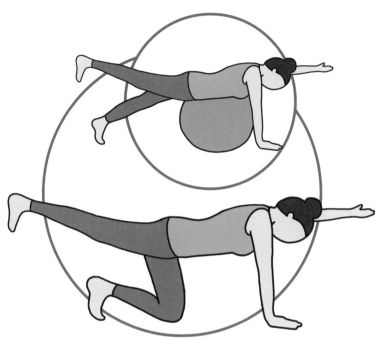

BIRD DOG POSE

This can be performed on your hands and knees or with an exercise ball. Looking down at the floor, lift your left leg and foot and your right arm at the same time; hold for one to two seconds. Return to starting position and raise the opposite arm and leg.

Repeat 20 times.

Strengthens: Posture and lower back.

BRIDGE

Lie on your back, knees bent and feet flat on the floor. Raise your hips toward the ceiling while your shoulder and upper back remain on the floor. Hold for two to three seconds, and then lower yourself back onto the floor.

Repeat 10–20 times.

Strengthens: Pelvic floor, glutes, and the core.

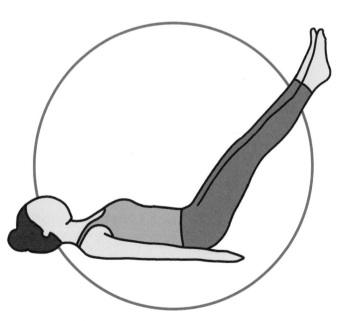

LEG LIFTS

Lie flat on your back with your hands either at your side or behind your neck, whichever is most comfortable. Pressing your lower back to the floor, raise your legs 90 degrees off the floor; hold for one to two seconds. Exhale and slowly lower your legs back to the ground.

Repeat 10 times.

Strengthens: Pelvic floor and abdominal muscles.

WARNING: Before doing any exercise, consult with your health-care provider to ensure a specific exercise is right for you and your recovery.

C-SECTION RECOVERY

GETTING STARTED

The who, what, and when of the process of returning to your former self after a C-section.

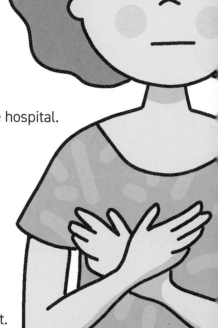

QUICK TIP

A belly band can be a **LIFESAVER!** You don't realize how much you use your abs, from pooping and simply moving to, God forbid, coughing or sneezing.

WHAT IS IT?

C-SECTION/CESAREAN: A major surgery where a cut is made through the abdominal wall and uterus to deliver a baby. Its recovery time is longer than that of a vaginal birth.

There are two types of incisions that can be used for a C-section: midline and bikini. It tends to take longer to recover from a vertical cut. As you heal, the surgical area may feel a bit numb. Most people regain all sensation, but if your numbness continues, speak to your doctor, who will determine whether there is some nerve damage.

GENERAL RECOVERY TIME

6–8 WEEKS

Recovery time can vary from individual to individual.

WHILE IN THE HOSPITAL

After a Cesarean, you are likely to spend two to four days in the hospital. During this time, the hospital staff will:

- Help with pain management.
- Make sure you are eating and drinking enough.
- Help you begin to get mobile.
- Help you with breastfeeding, if you choose to do it.
- Clean and dress your wound.
- Help you with going to the bathroom.
- Provide wound-care information and pain management.

TIPS FOR RECOVERY

When you return home, here are some things to do to help your recovery:

- Try to rest as much as possible.

- Avoid heavy lifting: nothing heavier than your baby.

- Avoid twisting your body or movement that puts pressure on the wound.

- Keep the incision clean and dry.

- Follow your pain-management plan.

- Try a heating pad (on low) or warm washcloth to ease pain around your belly.

- When sneezing, coughing, or laughing, hold your belly.

- No sex during the recovery period.

- Create a support system, if you haven't already done it, for meals, laundry, etc.

- Make an effort to get some exercise; try walking around a little.

TIPS FOR CARING FOR YOUR INCISION

SHOWERING: You should be able to take a shower (confirm with your doctor), letting the water run down over the wound.

WASHING: Use a mild soap when cleaning the wound. Do not scrub. Pat dry.

BATHING: Do not soak in a tub or hot tub or swim until your doctor approves it.

RELIEVING PAIN: Check with your doctor, but you may be able to use ibuprofen or acetaminophen.

AVOIDING INFECTION: Keep an eye out for signs of infections, for example:

- Your wound is red and swollen.
- Your wound is hot to the touch.
- Your wound is leaking.
- You have a fever.
- Your pain is getting worse.
- You are experiencing bleeding.

Mommy Hack

BATHROOM TIP

Wearing pants with a drawstring can be helpful, as you can hold the string in your mouth while using your hands to lift yourself off the toilet. Or call your partner.

C-SECTION SCAR CARE

WHAT TO KNOW

Everyone is different. Some people tend to scar more than others, but proper care of your incision is important. Consult your health-care provider as to the right treatment for you.

WHAT IS IT?

A C-section delivery can lead to some significant scarring. Some scars fade over time; others may become thick, red, and bulge.

Mommy Hack

Compression garments are a good way to protect your C-section scar as it heals. They come in tights, shorts, and corsets.

TIPS FOR TREATING EXISTING SCARS

SILICONE TREATMENT: Silicone gel or strips help reduce the appearance of scars over time by hydrating the upper layer of skin. It helps produce a fibroblast and reduces collagen production, which can result in a softer, flatter scar.

STEROID INJECTIONS: Typically used for larger scars, steroids are injected directly into the scar tissue to help reduce itching and redness and to help flatten the scar.

LASER THERAPY: This technique can help soften or remove scars by removing the outer layer of skin or stimulating the production of new skin cells.

SCAR REVISION: This cosmetic surgical procedure reopens the scar in order to remove the scar tissue and allow the new cut to heal with less scarring.

TUMMY TUCK: An intense form of cosmetic surgery cuts away the scar, additional skin, and fat to improve the overall shape and appearance of the abdomen.

NOTE: Always speak to your health-care provider/professional about the risks involved and what procedures are safe and appropriate treatment for you and your condition.

TIPS FOR PREVENTING SCARRING

KEEP IT CLEAN: Proper care of your incision can prevent infection and help keep scarring to a minimum. When showering, let soapy water run over it. No scrubbing; pat dry.

STAY HYDRATED: Hydration helps the healing process.

DON'T STRESS THE INCISION: Avoid moving in ways, such as twisting, that overly stress the incision. Hold off exercise until your doctor gives you the green light.

EAT HEALTHY: A healthy diet is important; it gives the body everything it needs to heal.

OINTMENTS: Ask your doctor if they recommend any topical ointments.

AIR IT OUT: Allowing a wound to breathe—good air circulation—can promote healing; stick to loose-fitting clothing.

NO SUN: During the first six weeks, do not expose your scar to the sun. It can make the scar more visible. If you have to be in the sun, use a strong SPF sunblock.

ALCOHOL & CIGARETTES: It's best to avoid alcohol and cigarettes; they can impair the skin's natural healing ability and dehydrate cells.

SCAR MASSAGE

Cesarean deliveries affect several layers of tissue. As your scar heals, the layers can become stuck to each other, impairing movement.

Scar tissue massage helps to break up the adhesions and helps promote healing as well as improving the appearance of the scar. Only begin scar tissue massage after speaking with your health-care provider.

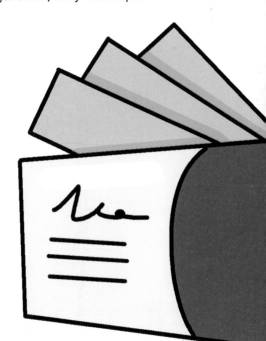

C-SECTION EXERCISES
WHAT TO DO AND WHEN

Here are some things that will help you get back in shape after a Cesarean.

GETTING STARTED

It's generally recommended that 24 hours after surgery, you start slowly moving around. This small amount of activity helps relieve gas pains, begin bowel movements, and prevent blood clots.

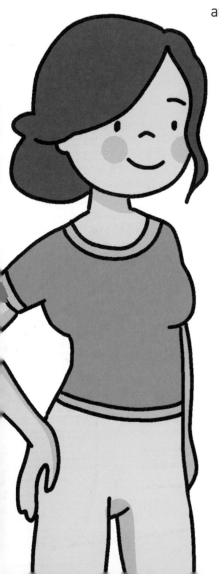

DAILY ACTIVITY

You should take it easy for the first couple of weeks. Check with your doctor to find out what activities are OK for you.

THINGS TO KNOW

LIFTING: Don't lift anything heavy for at least four to six weeks after surgery.

BATHING: Wait three weeks before taking a bath or using a hot tub.

STAIRS: Avoid stairs, if possible. If you have to take them, be careful, and go slowly.

DRIVING: Wait two weeks before you drive. Do not drive if using opioid pain medication, as this will make you drowsy.

SWIMMING: Wait six weeks before swimming.

WHAT EXERCISES TO START WITH

DEEP BREATHING: Begin by taking deep breaths. Breathe in and fill your lungs, and then slowly, on the count of four, breathe out fully. Repeat two to three times every half hour.

STRETCHING: You can begin light stretches of your arms, neck, shoulders, and legs, but do not put any pressure on your incision.

KEGEL EXERCISES: You can start Kegel exercises once your catheter is removed and you feel ready.

WALKING: Go slowly, but as soon as you can, get up and move around. Try to get in a little walking (maybe around the block a few times).

POSTURE: Practice good posture; sitting up straight, shoulders back can help strengthen your abdominal muscles.

GENERAL RECOMMENDATION

6–8 WEEKS REST
BEFORE BEGINNING EXERCISE

WHATS NEXT

At the six-week point, you will be seeing your doctor, who will see how you are healing. At that time, ask about an appropriate exercise routine. Find out what is OK and what is NOT for you.

If given the OK, you may begin low-impact postpartum exercises, but ease into abdominal exercises.

WARNING

Before doing any exercise, check with you health-care provider to make sure any specific exercise is right for your body and your specific recovery.

SEX
SEX AFTER DELIVERY

What to know and what to do when you are ready for sex.

QUICK TIP

PREGNANT?
Even if you have not started menstruating, and you are breastfeeding, you can still get pregnant. Consider birth control options!

OVERVIEW

When is the right time for sex after you give birth?

Actually, it is a completely personal, individual decision. No one can make that decision for you—nor should they!

Health-care practitioners generally agree that you should wait <u>a minimum</u> of:

4–6 WEEKS

<u>Or even more</u> . . . which seems reasonable, considering you may:

- Still be healing.
- Have vaginal tears.
- Have vaginal discharge and bleeding.
- Have had surgical repair done.
- Are overall fatigued.
- Be experiencing vaginal dryness.
- Have pain and soreness.
- Be experiencing low sex drive.

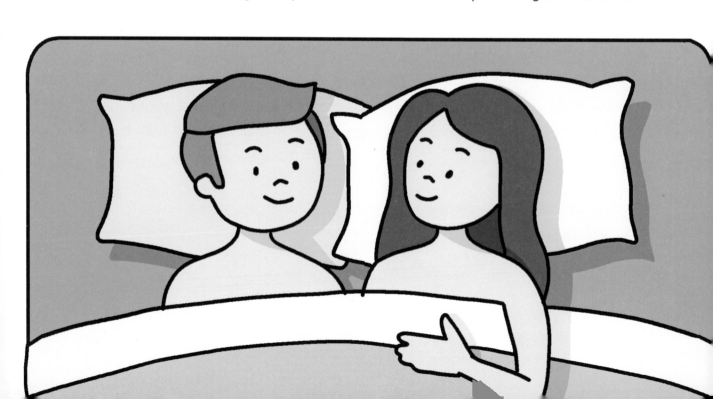

TALK, TALK, TALK

It's important to talk about sex. If either you or your partner is interested, don't hesitate to talk about how you feel—maybe you are not feeling sexy, or are afraid, or, if you are ready, what are you ready for?

WILL IT HURT?

YES, MAYBE:

Hormonal changes can leave your vagina dry and tender.

Breastfeeding can lower your libido.

Episiotomy or perineal tears can cause you to experience some pain during sex.

EASING SEX DISCOMFORT TIPS

PREPARE FOR PAIN

Taking steps before sex to minimize or eliminate pain can help:

· Empty your bladder.   · Take a warm bath.   · Take pain medication.

LUBE IT UP

If you are experiencing vaginal dryness, using lubricant can be helpful.

INTERCOURSE ALTERNATIVES

There are other ways—from oral sex to masturbation—to satisfy your partner and yourself without having vaginal sex. Look at it as an opportunity to try some new, fun things.

BE PATIENT

Make time to have sex when you are not too tired. If you are concerned, take it slow.

GOING DEEP

To start, you might want to manage the level of penetration. Choose a position that limits it—for example, spooning or woman on top.

JUST NOT INTERESTED

That is perfectly fine; you will be ready when you are ready. Until then, remember intimacy is not just sex; you can show affection and that you care in other ways, but it is very important to demonstrate your love.

SCARED SHITLESS
POSTPARTUM POO & PEE

We're going to be honest: it hurts and it really sucks, but knowing what to expect can help you be better prepared to minimize the pain.

QUICK TIP
Be careful going to the bathroom right after delivery—you might be light-headed, so it is wise to have some help.

OVERVIEW

Whether you had a vaginal or Cesarean delivery, being concerned about peeing and pooing after delivery is normal.

Normally your first poo and pee happen

FIRST POO: 3–5 DAYS

FIRST PEE: 1–2 HOURS

Like all things with pregnancy, different people will experience their first postpartum poo and pee differently and it may be sooner.

WHY IS IT HAPPENING?

Going to the bathroom can be affected by:

CONTRACTIONS: Mild contractions will continue after delivery as your uterus shrinks back to its normal size. These contractions cause bowel movements.

PELVIC FLOOR: Giving birth stretches the muscles of your pelvic floor. Loosening these muscles can cause constipation and a leaky bladder.

HORMONES: Hormones affect your bowel movement. They can cause constipation, diarrhea, and urinary incontinence.

HEMORRHOIDS: These swollen veins of the rectum and anus can make bowel movements painful and lead to constipation.

MEDICAL INTERVENTIONS: Procedures such as a vaginal tear, episiotomy, or Cesarean can cause bowel and urinary incontinence.

FIRST POOP CONCERNS

- Constipation
- Diarrhea
- Hemorrhoids
- Fecal incontinence

TIPS FOR POOPING

HYDRATE: Drink plenty of water, eight glasses a day.

TAKE STOOL SOFTENER: It can help ease constipation.

GET MOVING: Walking helps get bowels moving.

EAT HEALTHY: Eat whole grains, fruits, veggies, lots of fiber.

TAKE A SITZ BATH: Take sitz baths and use padsicles.

DO KEGEL EXERCISES: Strengthening the pelvic floor muscles.

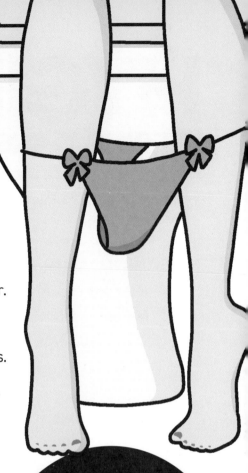

FIRST PEE CONCERNS

- Pain and burning
- Nerve damage
- Difficulty peeing
- Urinary incontinence

TIPS FOR PEEING

Peeing after childbirth can be quite painful! Here are some tips and techniques to help minimize the pain:

PERI BOTTLE: A peri bottle is a container that is filled with warm water and, while peeing, you spray on the area to dilute the urine, helping to decrease the pain and wash the area.

Mommy Hack

Consider investing in several peri bottles that you can keep in the bathroom and in your purse and car in case you have to go while running around.

MEDICATION: Take a doctor-recommended pain medication that can help reduce the swelling and alleviate pain. Placing a cold pack or a padsicle on the sore area for 10 to 20 minutes at a time may also help.

NUMBING SPRAY: Use a pain-relief spray to numb the area.

PEE IN THE BATH OR SHOWER: You can try turning on the shower and peeing while the warm water runs over you. You can also try peeing in a bath or sitz bath.

HYGIENE
KEEPING THINGS CLEAN DOWN THERE

Good hygiene during and after the birth of your baby is important; it can help reduce discomfort and prevent infections. Here are some things you should know.

CLEANING YOUR PRIVATE PARTS

After delivery, keeping yourself clean is important. There are several things you will want to clean your privates of:

- **VAGINAL DISCHARGE:** As your body sheds the remains of the mucous membrane that lines the uterus, you will experience vaginal discharge, which is a combination of blood and mucous.
- **URINE**
- **POOP**

BLEEDING

After delivery, for the next couple days, you will experience some heavy bleeding. It can be two to three times as bad as your worst period. That is followed by a lighter discharge that lasts for around four to six weeks.

INFECTION

Watch for signs of infection, which include:

- Fever or chills
- Excessive bleeding (soaking a pad an hour)
- Losing consciousness
- Bad smelling vaginal discharge
- Redness or swelling
- Difficulty peeing
- Sudden weakness
- Headaches
- Abdominal pain
- Rapid heartbeat

NOTE: If you experience any of these symptoms, call your doctor immediately.

TIPS FOR GOOD HYGIENE

KEEP THE PERINEUM CLEAN

Keeping the area between your vagina and rectum clean is important.

WASH YOUR HANDS

Every time you go to the bathroom or change your pad, be sure to wash your hands before and after.

CHANGE PADS FREQUENTLY

Change your sanitary pad often! You want to change it four to six times a day and definitely change it every time you go number two.

USE A SQUIRT BOTTLE

Using a squirt bottle or peri bottle can be very helpful when cleaning yourself after going to the bathroom. Squirt warm water from front to back and pat dry—do not rub.

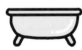

USE A BIDET

Using a bidet, if you have one, to clean your privates can be more convenient than showering.

TAKE A SITZ BATH

Soaking in a sitz tub can also help keep things clean and soothe soreness, especially after vaginal deliveries.

BLOW DRY

Some new moms use a hair dryer on the cool setting to dry their private parts to avoid touching that very sensitive area.

DO NOT USE TAMPONS

Absolutely no tampons (they can create infections) until your doctor tells you it is OK.

SLEEP
WHAT IS THAT?

One of the areas of your life that will be significantly impacted by your new bundle of joy is sleep.

OVERVIEW

SLEEP—oh glorious sleep!

I'm sorry to say that sleep generally can be really challenging in those first months when you have to wake up every couple of hours to feed baby. That and the stress of new parenthood can make it tough to fall asleep and stay asleep.

For some, sleep is even more challenging because they are experiencing postpartum insomnia.

POSTPARTUM INSOMNIA

A somewhat common problem whereby some moms are consistently unable to fall asleep or stay asleep following the birth of their baby.

CAUSES

- Anemia
- Mood disorders
- Hormonal changes
- Anxiety
- Physical discomfort
- Sleep schedule changes

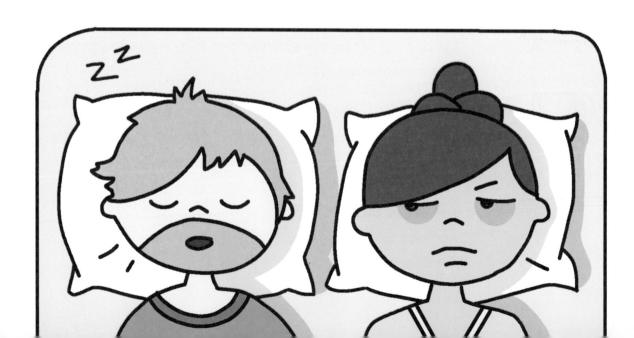

TIPS TO HELP YOU GET SOME ZZZZs

SLEEP WHEN BABY SLEEPS

If you are seriously running low on sleep, it's time to nap when baby sleeps. It is not time to try to get in those household chores—they can wait.

SLEEP ROUTINE

Try and stick to a regular sleep routine.

SLEEP ENVIRONMENT

Create an environment that is best for falling asleep. Keep the room cool and dark. Turn off any electronics that might interfere with your sleep. Consider buying pillows, a mattress, or blankets that feel good to you.

DE-STRESS

Finding ways to relieve or reduce stress can significantly improve your sleep—ask your doctor for recommendations.

WORK TOGETHER

Sharing the chores and nights is really helpful. If you need to, pump ahead of time so your partner can take over some of the night feeding.

DISCONNECT

Cutting screen time at night is very helpful. Screens from your phone, desktop, or other digital devices activate your brain, making it difficult to sleep.

EXERCISE

Getting daily exercise improves sleep. Even going for a daily walk has benefits, but avoid exercising right before you go to bed.

LIMIT CAFFEINE & ALCOHOL

Caffeine, nicotine, and alcohol interfere with the natural sleep process—so limit it.

EXTRA SUPPORT

Ask for a little help—maybe shopping or caring for baby—from your family or friends while you take a little nap.

PADSICLES
AHHHHH SOME COOL RELIEF!

Taking care of yourself, especially your vaginal area, is a priority during postpartum. Here is what you need to know about giving that extra TLC to your lady parts.

WHAT IS IT?

PADSICLE: Also called a cooling pad, it is a specially prepared sanitary napkin that is placed in the freezer to chill and used to soothe pain and encourage healing after a vaginal delivery. In essence, padsicles are an alternative to an icepack. They can also be covered with additional healing ingredients.

WHY USE IT?

After vaginal delivery, there is a lot of swelling, pain, bruising, and soreness; the padsicle helps ease that postpartum discomfort.

WHEN TO MAKE THEM

It's recommended that you create a bunch of padsicles during the last month of your pregnancy. That way you won't have to bother making them while you are recovering.

HOW TO USE

Take the padsicle out of the freezer and let it thaw for a couple minutes.

Two options:

1. Place it in your underwear as you would a regular pad, or place it on a towel and sit on it. Depending on how much witch hazel you use, you may prefer the towel, since the pad might leak if it's heavily saturated.

2. Wear the padsicle inside an adult diaper. This gives added protection if your postpartum flow is heavy.

WHAT YOU WILL NEED:

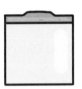

Plastic bag

Maxi sanitary
napkin or pads
(chlorine-free)

Witch hazel
without alcohol

100% pure
lavender oil

100% pure unscented
organic aloe vera gel

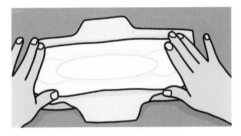

STEP 1:

Unwrap a sanitary napkin or pad; lay it out flat and unfold the paper tabs from the napkin so it is fully open. Leave the back wrapper attached.

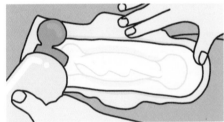

STEP 2:

Generously apply the aloe vera gel to the napkin. Spread the gel over the whole pad with a clean finger or spoon. You will want to cover as much of the surface as you can, but not the side wings.

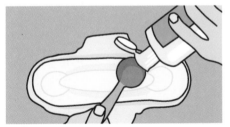

STEP 3:

Apply a second layer of alcohol-free witch hazel down the middle of the pad—two to three tablespoons—you want it wet, not soaked.

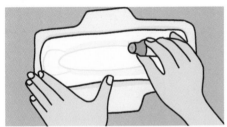

STEP 4: (Optional)

Apply several drops of lavender oil onto the pad.

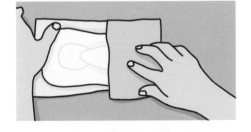

STEP 5:

Gently fold the pad and put in a plastic bag and place in the freezer for at least an hour.

SITZ BATH
TIME FOR A SOAK

The healing process after childbirth is another of those less-than-thrilling parts of having a baby. A sitz bath might just be one of the more pleasurable activities.

WHAT IS IT?

SITZ BATH: A treatment that can relieve the pain and itching that comes from sore, swollen skin, stitches, and hemorrhoids. To take a sitz bath, you sit in warm, shallow water to cleanse the space between the anus and the vulva.

WHAT IT DOES

- Promotes healing by relaxing the muscles and increasing blood flow to the area.
- Helps keep the area clean to prevent infection.
- Reduces soreness and swelling.
- Relieves itching.

SITZ BATH METHODS

METHOD 1: THE BATHTUB

Make sure the bathtub is clean! You don't want there to be any bacteria that might cause an infection.

Fill the tub with two to four inches of warm water (not hot) to cover your whole vagina. You might add any substances your doctor recommends to the bath.

Soak for 15 to 20 minutes three to four times a day. If possible, bend your knees or dangle your legs over the side of the tub.

Pat yourself dry using a clean cotton towel. Do not rub the area, as it may cause pain or irritation. Clean the bathtub thoroughly.

SITZ BATH METHODS

METHOD 2: A SITZ BATH KIT

This is a small basin that rests on top of the toilet so that you can sit on it.

 STEP 1 Make sure the basin is clean. You don't want any bacteria that might cause an infection. (Many kits come with cleaning instructions.)

 STEP 2 Fill with warm water (not hot), adding any substances your doctor recommends to the bath. It should contain enough water to cover your vaginal area.

 STEP 3 Place the sitz bath on the toilet as instructed, and test to make sure it is secure. Lower yourself carefully onto the seat; don't worry about overflow, as the tub is designed with a notch to spill any overflow into the toilet.

 STEP 4 Soak for 15 to 20 minutes, three to four times a day.

 STEP 5 Pat yourself dry using a clean cotton towel. Do not rub the area, as it may cause pain or irritation. Clean the basin thoroughly.

COMMON SITZ ADD-INS

- Epsom salts
- Witch hazel
- Baking soda
- Sea salt (non-iodized)
- Vinegar
- Povidone-iodine

NOTE: Always speak to your health-care provider/professional about any risks involved and what is safe and right for you and your pregnancy.

Safety is
no accident.

SAFETY

Some things to think about when it comes to baby's and your safety.

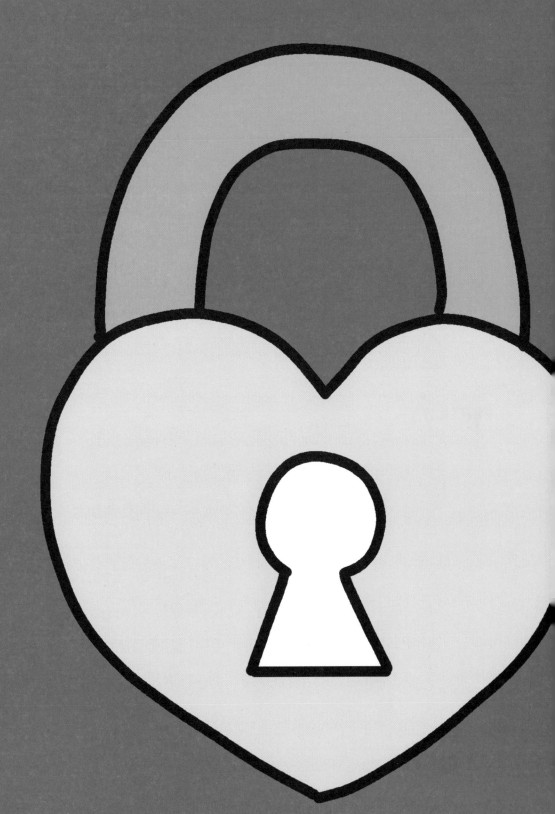

HAVING A BABY
AGE AND RISK

Having a baby at an older age may have more risk of complications than when you are younger, but ultimately the perfect time to get pregnant is when you feel it's right for you.

OVERVIEW

Many things go into the decision to get pregnant, from emotional readiness to financial security, from being in a stable relationship to your career. Women in the United States are increasingly delaying pregnancy into their thirties and beyond. With the increased age comes increased risk and more things to consider.

OPTIMAL AGE

Generally, it is agreed that the optimal time for a woman to have a positive outcome for both baby and mother is if she becomes pregnant when she is in her late twenties to early thirties.

FERTILITY

All women are born with a specific number of eggs, and over time, as she ages, the quality and quantity of the eggs decline.

To Start with:	1–2 Million Eggs
Puberty:	300–500 Thousand Eggs
Early 20s:	150–300 Thousand Eggs
Early 30s:	20–25 Thousand Eggs
Early 40s:	5–10 Thousand Eggs
Menopause:	0–1,000 Eggs

This can impact her ability to get pregnant and also comes with a greater chance of complications.

COMPLICATIONS

Starting at around age 35, the risk of complications, such as the following, increase:

- Gestational diabetes
- High blood pressure
- Miscarriage or stillbirth
- Multiple births
- Premature delivery
- Chromosomal abnormalities
- Cesarean delivery
- Blockages of the fallopian tubes
- Decreased fertility
- Heavy bleeding postdelivery

GETTING A LITTLE HELP

Technology has come a long way. If you are thinking of getting pregnant, and you are over 35, and have been trying for more than six months, you should speak to your doctor about:

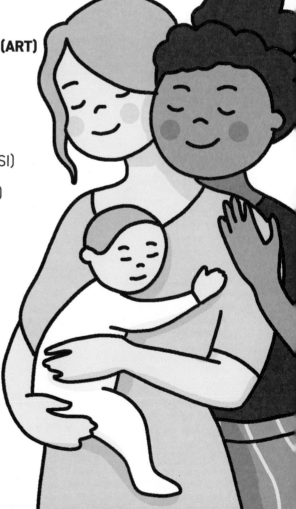

ASSISTED REPRODUCTIVE TECHNOLOGIES (ART)

These are technologies that help a woman conceive; among them are:

- In vitro fertilization (IVF)
- Intracytoplasmic sperm injection (ICSI)
- Gamete intrafallopian transfer (GIFT)
- Zygote intrafallopian transfer (ZIFT)

OLDER MEN

A man's fertility also declines with age, but this process doesn't start until around age 40. At this point, men have lower semen volume and sperm count than when they were young, and those they have aren't great swimmers.

CAUTION
PREGNANCY NO-NOs

Once you become pregnant, there are some things you should avoid to protect the health of your baby. Here is a list of what to be aware of.

THINGS TO AVOID DURING PREGNANCY

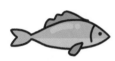

CERTAIN FOODS

There are many things to be careful of or to avoid when you are pregnant; among these are certain foods (refer to the No-No Foods page).

MEDICATIONS

Some medications can be harmful to your baby. Before taking any medication, prescription or over-the-counter, speak to your doctor.

HIGH HEELS

During pregnancy, your center of gravity shifts and can make you unsteady; high heels increase the risk of a fall.

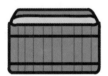

HOT TUBS & SAUNAS

Avoid hot tubs, saunas, steam rooms, hot yoga, or anything that elevates your body temperature, as it can be harmful to the baby.

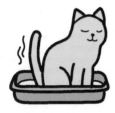

KITTY LITTER

Cat feces can carry toxoplasmosis, a parasitic disease. If you have a kitty, have someone else change the litter or wear gloves.

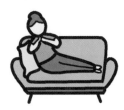

STAYING STATIONARY

Avoid standing or sitting in the same position for extended periods of time. It can cause many issues, from swollen ankles to poor blood circulation.

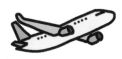

AIR TRAVEL

It is generally recommended that you not fly after 36 weeks, domestically, and 32 weeks, internationally, as long as you have a healthy pregnancy. Air travel may not be recommended for individuals who have certain or specific medical or obstetric conditions. (Consult with your health-care provider.)

X-RAYS

Avoid them, especially abdominal X-rays, while you are pregnant, unless the risk of not having one outweighs the risk of radiation. (Consult your health-care provider.)

AMUSEMENT PARK RIDES

Riding on certain attractions that are jarring or stop suddenly can cause the placenta to detach from the uterus.

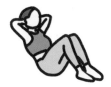

CERTAIN EXERCISES

Avoid exercises that involve bouncing, leaping, jumping, jerking, or require sudden changes in direction, as well as abdominal exercises like sit-ups.

HEAVY LIFTING

Lifting heavy objects could cause preterm labor.

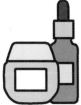

BEAUTY TREATMENTS

Occasional nail polish is generally considered safe. Use acetone-free nail polish remover. Avoid Botox injections, chemical peels, tanning beds, whitening stripes, self-tanners, and products containing retinoids, toluene, phthalates, formaldehyde, or hydroquinone. Some women delay using hair dyes until after 12 weeks of pregnancy. Consult your health-care provider.

ENVIRONMENTAL HAZARDS

THE HIDDEN HAZARDS

Our world is full of chemicals that can potentially harm your baby. Here is what they are and ways to try to avoid them.

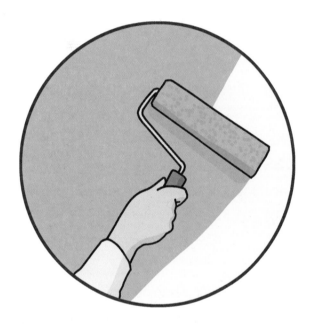

PAINT & SOLVENTS

Many paints contain toxic solvents and chemicals that can be very harmful if you inhale too much of them. Harmful solvents can be found in paint strippers, thinners, varnish, and other household products.

TIPS:

- Use low or zero VOC (volatile organic compounds) paints.
- Make sure you have good ventilation.
- Wear a N95 or equivalent mask.
- Wear gloves and avoid contact with skin.

HOUSEHOLD PRODUCTS

Cleaning products contain lots of chemicals that can harm you and your baby—chemicals like bisphenol A (BPA) and phthalates.

TIPS:

- Reduce consumption of processed foods.
- Eat and drink from phthalate-free plastics.
- Use microwave-safe cookware.
- Use nontoxic cleaning products or make your own.
- Use in well-ventilated spaces.

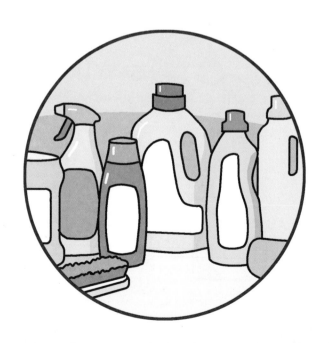

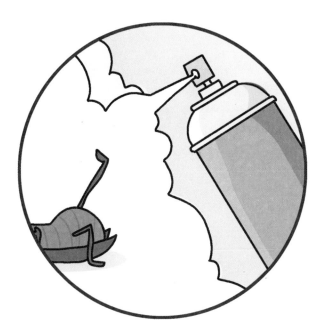

PESTICIDES & INSECT REPELLENTS

Exposure to pesticides may come from eating pesticide-contaminated food or using pesticides in the home, garden, or on pets. Insect repellents may contain the chemical DEET, which is also harmful to baby.

TIPS:

· Avoid using chemical tick and flea collars or dips.
· Avoid using pesticides indoors and outside.
· Wash food thoroughly before eating it.
· Avoid lawn chemicals and fertilizers.

CONSTRUCTION

Many new and old building materials contain dangerous chemicals, which can include dust, mold, lead, asbestos, and fumes.

TIPS:

· Avoid construction sites.
· Seal off the part of the house under construction.
· Remove any residual dust.
· Ventilate the area.

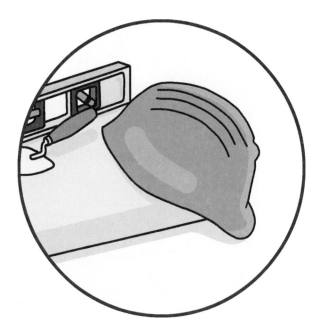

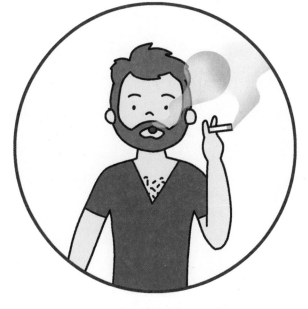

SECONDHAND SMOKE

Secondhand smoke can be just as bad as smoking. It exposes baby to numerous harmful chemicals.

TIPS:

· Avoid being around anyone who is smoking.
· Smokers' clothing should be avoided until clean.
· After being around smoke, wash your hands and face before touching your baby.
· If around smokers, do it in a well-ventilated area.

AIR TRAVEL
WHEN YOU GOTTA GO, YOU GOTTA GO

Sometimes not traveling is not an option. If you must travel, here are some things to consider before you go.

IS TRAVEL SAFE?

Generally, air travel is considered safe during a healthy pregnancy with no complications up until 36 weeks when flying domestically and 32 weeks when flying internationally.

Before going:

· Check with your health-care provider to be certain that flying is safe for you.

· Check your airline's policies.

HAVE A PLAN

Just in case an emergency arises while you are away, make sure you have the name of a medical facility where you can get obstetric care. Pack a copy of your medical records and the name and contact information of your doctor in your carry-on, in case you go into labor mid-flight.

THE BEST TIME TO FLY

The best time to take to the skies might be during the second trimester, when the pregnancy risks are typically at their lowest. Ultimately, when to fly will depend on how you are feeling at the time.

GET CLEARED

If you are going to be traveling, be sure to speak to your doctor before you go to ensure that it's safe for you. You might ask them about:

· Compression socks

· Nausea remedies

· Diarrhea remedies

TIPS FOR FLYING

BUCKLE UP

Keep your seatbelt buckled and fastened under your belly, low on the hips.

PRENATAL VITAMINS

Make sure you have enough vitamins for the trip.

CLOTHING

Wear a loose, comfortable outfit and shoes, and check with your doctor about wearing compression socks.

Mommy Hack

Wearing compression socks while on the plane will help promote circulation and reduce swelling.

SNACKS

Have snacks ready and easily accessible.

GAS

Avoid eating or drinking anything that might give you gas—beans, broccoli, cabbage, and carbonated drinks.

GET UP AND MOVE

Taking a walk every half hour will help promote circulation. If you must remain seated, periodically flex your ankles and legs.

HYDRATE

Airplanes are notoriously dry, so drink plenty of water to stay hydrated.

YOUR SEAT

Try to book an aisle seat so you don't have to climb over people to get out.

BEAUTY

KEEP THE GLOW, LOSE THE ____

Becoming pregnant means lots of changes. Your beauty regimen may need a slight adjustment in order to best take care of you and your baby.

OVERVIEW

Most over-the-counter cosmetic products are safe, but there are a few things you should be aware of and some things it might be best to avoid during pregnancy.

CHEMICALS OF CONCERN

While evidence-based data on the effects of cosmetic ingredients on pregnant women is limited, animal-based data is available. This research suggests that there are certain chemicals used in cosmetic products that might affect your pregnancy and be worth trying to avoid.

Chemicals to watch for:

- Retinoids
- High doses of salicylic acid
- Hydroquinone
- Phthalates
- Formaldehyde
- Parabens
- Bisphenol A
- Lead
- Tetracycline

- Oxybenzone
- Borneol
- Diazolidine urea
- Hydroxymethylglycinate
- Imidazolidine urea
- Triclosan
- Fragrance
- Toluene

These chemicals can be found in many cosmetic products, from acne treatments, peels, and sunscreens to lipsticks, foundations, and skin lighteners.

ALTERNATIVES

Look for products that are all-natural, nontoxic, hypoallergenic, and fragrance-free.

GET YOUR FREE SAFE BEAUTY LIST

Scan the QR code to easily get our recommendations for some of the best beauty products that are safe for you and baby.

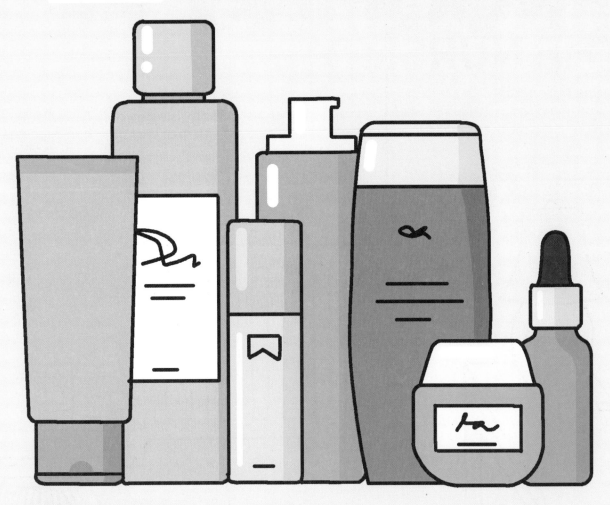

AVOID

- Chemical peels
- Self tanners
- Tanning beds
- Retinoid products
- Whitening stripes
- Botox injections

Occasional nail polish use is generally considered safe. However, try using nail polishes listed as "3-free" or "7-free" that do not contain products that may be harmful in pregnancy, and use only acetone-free nail polish remover. If you do go to a nail salon, make sure it's well-ventilated. Some women even delay coloring their hair until after 12 weeks of pregnancy.

NOTE: Always speak to your health-care provider and dermatologist to get their advice on what skin-care products are safe and right for you and your pregnancy.

CHILD-PROOFING
THE NURSERY

SMOKE DETECTOR
Install and test it regularly. Be sure to replace the batteries at least once a year.

ANCHOR FURNITURE
Anchor dressers and bookshelves to walls with braces to prevent them from toppling over onto your child. Keep toddlers from climbing up open dresser drawers by securing them with childproof locks.

GATES
Prevent late-night walkabouts by installing a baby gate or door with handle covers to prevent toddlers from opening the door.

OUTLETS
Put plastic outlet protectors over all unused electrical outlets.

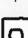
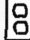

VENTING
Keep your baby from overheating, which is a known risk factor associated with SIDS; never place a crib next to a heater or in an area of direct sunlight.

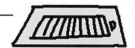

MATTRESS | BEDDING
Must be firm and fit the crib properly. There should be no more than two fingers' width of space between the side of the mattress and the crib frame. Use only a fitted sheet and fitted water-resistant mattress cover.

RUGS
Place nonslip pads under all area rugs.

Scan this QR code to order the
#1 Bestselling Book:
THE SIMPLEST BABY BOOK IN THE WORLD
to get more information on childproofing your home

Don't hang anything, for example, mirrors and large frames, over the crib. They could fall and injure your baby.

MOBILES
Remove crib mobiles, especially once your child can stand.

Position crib away from windows and other furniture in case your child attempts to climb out of the crib. Install window stops to prevent windows from opening more than a few inches. Remove or tie up window blind cords, as they pose a strangulation hazard.

No blankets, pillows, bumpers, or plush toys should be placed in the crib. These items all pose a risk of suffocation or entrapment and should never be used in a baby's crib.

CRIBS
Should be sturdy with fixed sides and slats spaced no more than 2 3/8 inches apart and made of eco-friendly, sustainable materials and nontoxic paint. Headboards should not have decorative cutouts or embellishments that clothing could catch on.

ROCKER | GLIDER
Protect little toes and fingers by choosing a glider with a stop-lock mechanism that prevents the chair from gliding when not in use, and be sure that all gears are encased and out of reach.

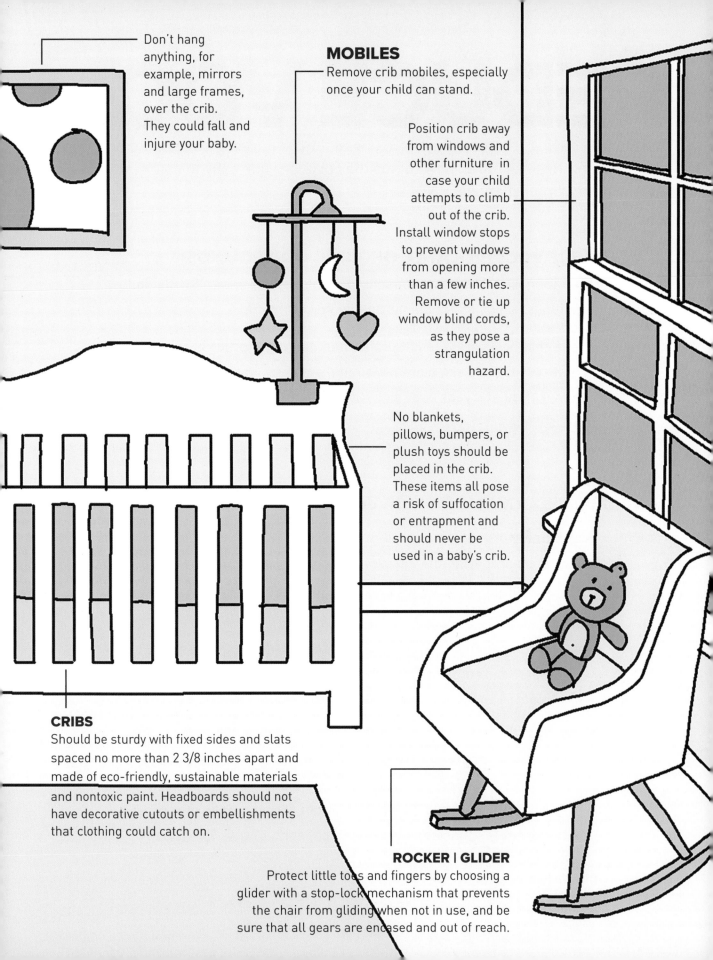

REDUCE VOCs

As you purchase all the fun items you'll need for the nursery, you should be aware that many of these beautiful new things may expose your baby to some potentially harmful chemicals: VOCs.

WHAT ARE VOCs (VOLATILE ORGANIC COMPOUNDS)?

They are gases that many household items give off under normal indoor conditions, which affect the air quality in your home.

These chemicals are a result of the manufacturing process and can be found in mattresses, carpets, paints, clothing, and even toys. They create fumes that can make you and your baby sick. Over time these chemicals dissipate, but it takes a while.

TIPS TO REDUCE THE RISK OF VOCs

Start Early

Start preparing the nursery early so that you can let the room air out for a month before your little bundle of joy arrives.

Paint

When painting the nursery, choose ultra-low-VOC, zero-VOC, or water-based paints. You should still leave ample time for ventilating the room.

Flooring

Flooring, especially carpet, can emit lots of VOCs, depending on what you use. Carpet made from natural, VOC-free materials, such as wool, cotton, sisal, or jute, are better choices than carpets made of synthetic materials. Consider wood, bamboo, cork, or a simple area rug.

High-Efficiency Air Purifier
These filters help purify the air and can remove 99.97 percent particles bigger than 0.3 micron in diameter.

PAINTING
Replace solvent-based paints with low-VOC or zero-VOC paints.

BEDDING
Hypoallergenic bedding and mattress can be used to curtail contaminants.

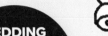

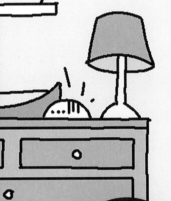

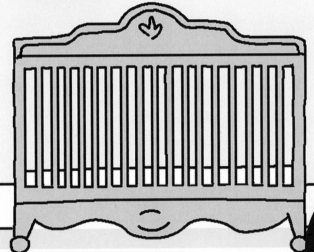

UNSCENTED
Avoid the use of scented items, like candles, dryer sheets, air fresheners, etc.

FURNITURE
Especially when made of pressed wood and plastics, furniture is the source of a variety of VOCs. Look for items that are Greenguard certified.

CARPET
Keep carpet in your nursery to a minimum, as carpet traps dust mites, pollen, animal dander, and mold spores and can emit (or "off-gas") harmful VOCs.

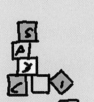

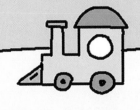

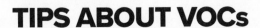

TIPS ABOUT VOCs

You can never
know too much to
learn something new.

HEALTH
& CONCERNS

Having a baby is complicated, and there are lots of things you need to know. These are some of the top issues and concerns you should be aware of.

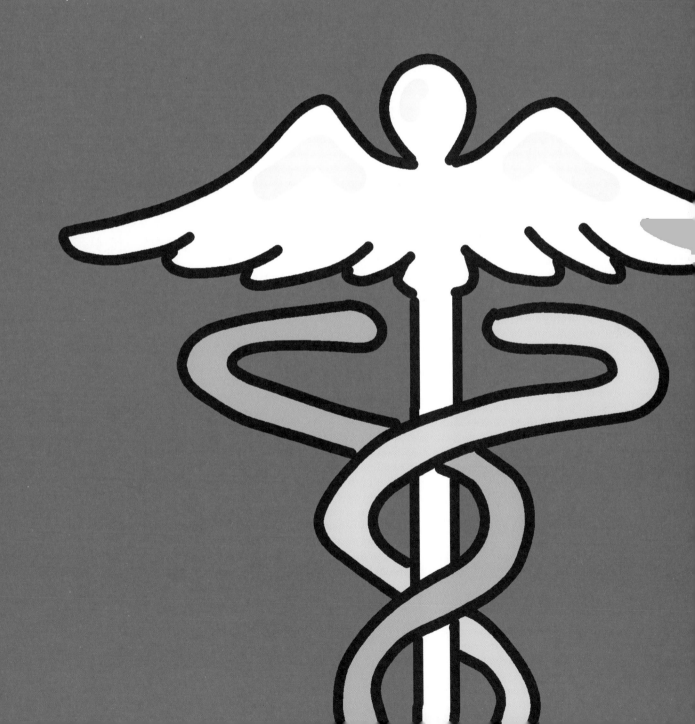

PRENATAL SCREENING
GETTING STARTED

WHAT IS IT?

PRENATAL SCREENING: Testing to identify whether your baby is likely to have certain genetic disorders and birth defects. Screening is not necessarily definitive; if results show a potential genetic condition or a birth defect, it is likely you will be given the option to have additional diagnostic testing done to confirm a potential disorder.

HOW IS IT DONE?

The types of prenatal testing are:

1. Blood tests   2. Ultrasound   3. Prenatal cell-free DNA screening

WHEN IS IT DONE?

FIRST TRIMESTER:

During your first trimester doctor visit, you'll have a Nuchal translucency screening: an ultrasound that is done between 10 and 13 weeks that measures the thickness of tissue on the back of the fetus's neck. This provides information about the risk of Down syndrome and other genetic conditions.

SECOND TRIMESTER:

During your second trimester visit, you will likely be given another blood test; it screens for Down syndrome (trisomy 21), Edwards syndrome (trisomy 18), and neural tube defects.

Around 18 and 22 weeks you will likely have the anatomy ultrasound scan to evaluate any abnormalities in the brain, spine, heart, face, and limbs.

PRENATAL CELL-FREE DNA SCREENING:

A blood test for chromosomal problems in the DNA released from the placenta, found in the mother's bloodstream. Can be done as early as 10 weeks. Because it screens the sex chromosomes, it can also tell you the sex of the baby.

WHO GETS TESTED?

All pregnant women have the option of having prenatal testing. However, it is highly recommended that the testing be done on women:

- 35 and older.
- With a history or previous pregnancy with genetic issues.
- With abnormal ultrasound findings.

RISK

There is no risk to your baby. You may have a slight pain or bruising from where the needle was put in your arm to collect the blood.

RESULTS

NEGATIVE: Means your baby has a decreased risk of Down Syndrome or other common trisomy disorders, but it does not eliminate the possibility your baby may still have a disorder.

POSITIVE: Means there is an increased risk that your baby has one of these disorders.
These tests can't tell you for certain if your baby has a disorder; only further diagnostic testing can do that.

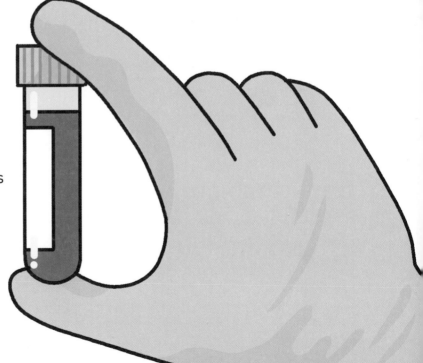

DIAGNOSTIC TESTING
CHECKING THINGS OUT

WHAT IS IT?

PRENATAL DIAGNOSTIC TESTING: The testing of the fetus before birth to determine if the baby has certain abnormalities.

WHEN IS IT DONE?

- If the results of a prenatal screening test come back positive.
- If abnormalities are found on the ultrasound.
- They may be offered to:
  - Women with a high-risk pregnancy.
  - Women 35 or older.
  - Women who had a previous pregnancy with birth defects.
  - Women with chronic diseases like lupus, high blood pressure, diabetes, etc.

WHAT ABNORMALITIES?

- Genetic conditions caused by an abnormal number of chromosomes (Down syndrome, Edward syndrome, for example).
- Inherited genetic disorders (sickle cell, cystic fibrosis, etc.)

TESTING METHODS

1. Chorionic villus sampling (CVS)
   - Transcervical
   - Transabdominal
2. Amniocentesis

NOTE: Always speak to your health-care provider/professional about the risks involved and if the procedure is safe and right for you and your pregnancy.

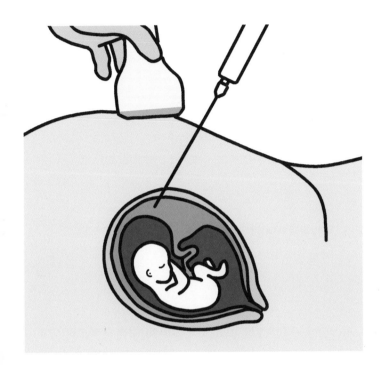

CHORIONIC VILLUS SAMPLING:

Tested at 10 to 13 weeks.

TRANSCERVICAL: A procedure where a catheter is inserted through the cervix into the placenta to obtain a tissue sample.

TRANSABDOMINAL: A procedure where a needle is inserted through the abdomen and uterus into the placenta to obtain a tissue sample.

RISK: Yes, slight risk of miscarriage.

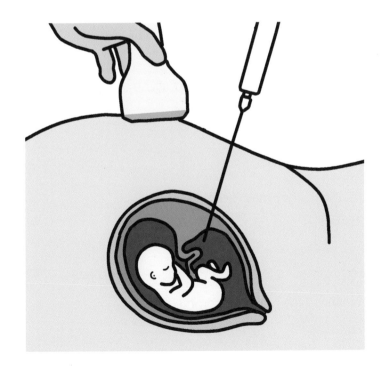

AMNIOCENTESIS:

Tested at 15 to 20 weeks.

A procedure in which a small amount of amniotic fluid is collected via a needle inserted through the abdomen into the amniotic sac. Cells in the fluid are tested for chromosomal disorders and genetic problems.

RISK: Yes, slight risk of miscarriage.

IMMUNIZATIONS
TO JAB OR NOT TO JAB?

If you are pregnant or planning to be, the specific vaccines you need are determined by your age, lifestyle, medical conditions, travel, and previous vaccinations.

RECOMMENDED VACCINES

The CDC recommends that pregnant women get three vaccines during pregnancy.

- **FLU VACCINE (inactivated)**

    It is recommended that all pregnant women get the flu vaccine to protect mom and baby, especially during the flu season.

- **TDAP VACCINE**

    Pregnant women are encouraged to get the Tdap vaccine during pregnancy, optimally between weeks 27 and 36 of their pregnancy, to protect them and their baby from whooping cough. If you don't get the vaccine during pregnancy, the CDC recommends that you get it immediately after giving birth.

- **COVID-19 VACCINE**

    The CDC recommends that pregnant people get the COVID-19 vaccine.

OTHER POSSIBLE VACCINATIONS

If your health-care provider thinks you are at risk, they may recommend:

- Hepatitis A & B
- Meningitis
- Pneumonia

If you are traveling and at risk of exposure to certain infections, please discuss with your health-care provider what additional vaccinations they might recommend.

VACCINES NOT TO GET

It is recommended that you NOT get certain vaccines during pregnancy:

- Tuberculosis (BCG)

- Human papillomavirus (HPV) vaccine

- Measles, Mumps, and Rubella (MMR) vaccine

- Flu vaccine (live) (Nasal Flu Vaccine)

- Chicken pox vaccine

- If you are traveling internationally, discuss with your health-care provider: Yellow Fever, Typhoid Fever, Japanese Encephalitis

BREASTFEEDING

Many vaccinations are safe for you and baby while you are breastfeeding, but consult with your health-care provider, letting them know you are breastfeeding to get their recommendations on any vaccinations and their safety for you and your baby.

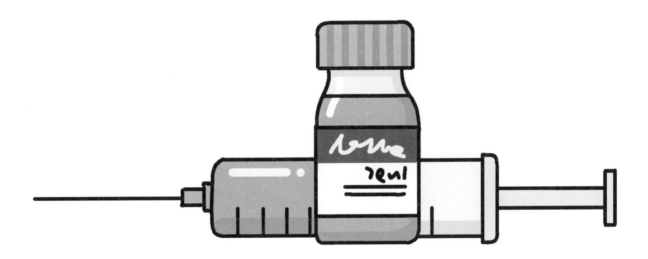

NOTE: Always speak to your health-care provider/professional about the risk involved and what is safe and right for you and your pregnancy.

MELASMA
SPOTS AND MORE SPOTS

The "mask of pregnancy" is normal and very common, albeit annoying.

WHAT IS IT?

MELASMA: A condition where the color-producing cells of the skin overproduce pigmentation. In pregnant woman it is called chloasma or the mask of pregnancy.

It appears as dark brown or grayish patches or spots on the face: usually the forehead, cheeks, chin, nose, or upper lip, although it can affect other parts of the body.

WHAT CAUSES IT?

You can thank the hormones estrogen and progesterone for these dark patches. Exposure to the sun can cause the condition to worsen. It tends to be worse in people with darker skin, which contains more skin pigmentation. Some skin-care products can also cause it to worsen.

WHEN DOES IT HAPPEN?

Typically, it develops in the second or third trimester, but it can happen at any time during pregnancy.

TREATMENT

There is no treatment for it; however, it usually fades several months after delivery.

RISK?

There is no risk to you or your baby.

TIPS FOR MINIMIZING MELASMA

DERMATOLOGIST:
Speak with your dermatologist for any recommendations.

SHADE:
Try and stay out of or limit your exposure to the sun. No tanning beds.

SKIN CARE:
Use gentle skin care and makeup products, as harsh ones can make melasma worse. Choose sensitive, fragrance-free products.

SUNSCREEN:
Wear sunscreen with an SPF 30 or above. Make sure the products are pregnancy-safe products that use zinc oxide, titanium dioxide, or mineral sunscreens.

COVER UP:
Wear loose-fitting clothes; cover exposed parts of the body. Wear a wide-brimmed hat to cover your face.

PATIENCE:
Once you have delivered your baby, things should begin to clear up in a few months.

YOUR TEETH
PROTECTING THOSE PEARLY WHITES

Being pregnant can affect your oral health; here is what you need to know to keep your mouth healthy.

OVERVIEW

The high levels of hormones in your body during pregnancy affect your oral health.

ORAL ISSUES
TEETH PROBLEMS:

1. TOOTH SENSITIVITY: Teeth can increase in sensitivity during pregnancy.

2. PERIODONTAL DISEASE: High levels of hormones may temporarily loosen the tissues and bones holding the teeth.

GUM PROBLEMS:

Sore, swollen, and bleeding gums can increase due to increased hormones.

1. GINGIVITIS (infection of the gums): Swelling and bleeding of the gums can be controlled by good dental hygiene.

2. PREGNANCY EPULIS OR PYOGENIC GRANULOMA: A localized swelling of the gums, which appears as a round, reddish growth on the gums. Also called pregnancy tumors, they are benign and usually disappear after the baby is born.

VOMITING:

The stomach acid from vomiting can damage the surface of teeth.

GAGGING:

Some women find that they tend to have a stronger gag reflex, and even brushing their teeth can trigger a gag reflex.

TIPS FOR ORAL HEALTH DURING PREGNANCY

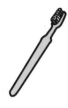

TOOTHBRUSH

Be sure to use an ADA-approved soft-bristle toothbrush. You may also try to get a small-head toothbrush if your gag reflex is creating a problem.

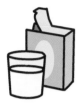

MORNING SICKNESS

After throwing up, don't brush your teeth right away. First rinse your mouth with one cup of water and a teaspoon of baking powder to prevent the stomach acid from eating away your teeth.

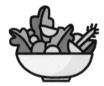

DIET

Eat a healthy diet, and keep sugary snacks to a minimum.

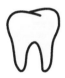

DENTIST

See your dentist regularly for cleaning and check-ups. Be sure to let your dentist know that you are pregnant. Postpone any elective dental procedures until after your baby is born.

BRUSHING

Brush twice a day with a fluoride toothpaste.

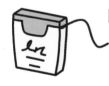

FLOSS

Floss once a day between teeth.

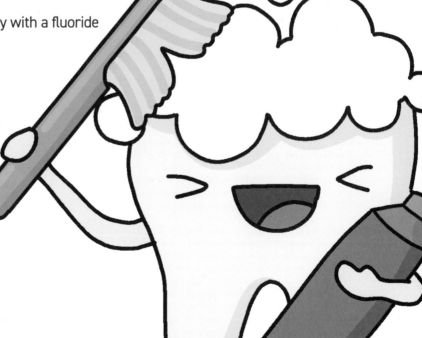

SICKLE CELL ANEMIA
SCD

WHAT IS IT?

SICKLE CELL ANEMIA (SCD): A hereditary blood disorder that causes the red blood cells to be misshaped into a crescent or sickle shape.

EFFECTS?

1. SHORTAGE OF RED BLOOD CELLS: The cells die early, resulting in a shortage of red blood cells which negatively affect the oxygen levels in the body, causing fatigue.

2. BLOCKED BLOOD FLOW: The affected sickle-shaped blood cells can slow and block blood flow.

CONCERNS FOR PREGNANCY

Women who have SCD can get worse during pregnancy, resulting in:

- Increased frequency and level of pain in organs and joints.

- Higher risk of premature birth.

- Increased infections and potential vision problems.

- Increased risk of miscarriage.

- Increased risk of anemia.

- High blood pressure.

- Preeclampsia.

- Increased risk of blood clots.

NOTE: Always speak to your health-care provider/professional about the risk involved and what is the safe and right treatment for you and your pregnancy.

WHAT TO DO?

With proper treatment and care, women with SCD can have a healthy pregnancy. But there are some things you should do to reduce the risk if you have SCD and are pregnant or planning on getting pregnant.

1 Speak with your health-care provider, and if you are of African or Hispanic ancestry, share that information, because these ethnicities have a higher risk of having the disease or carrying the genetic trait.

2 Get screened for the trait or disease.

3 Discuss having either chorionic villus sampling (CVS) or amniocentesis performed to find out if your baby has SCD.

4 Speak with your health-care provider about any medications you are taking for SCD.

5 Speak to your doctor about vaccinations and supplements that might be needed.

6 Avoid potential trigger of pain episodes, such as high altitudes, sudden temperature changes, dehydration, or intense exercise.

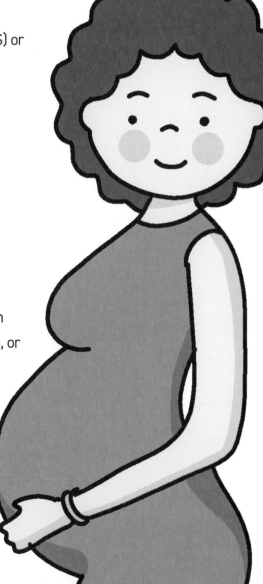

RH INCOMPATIBILITY
NOT MEANT TO BE TOGETHER

If you're considering becoming pregnant, it's a good idea to know your blood type and your Rh factor. With early detection and treatment, Rh incompatibility is almost completely preventable.

WHAT IS IT?

RH INCOMPATIBILITY: The Rh factor is a protein on the red blood cell. If you have a "positive" blood type, you are Rh positive, and if you have a "negative" blood type, you are Rh negative. Rh incompatibility is when a pregnant woman is Rh negative and the fetus is Rh positive.

Rh refers to the - or + you see after the letters; for example:

(AB-) is an Rh negative blood   (O+) is an Rh positive blood.

So if your baby has the same letters (AB) as you but a different Rh (- or +), then you could develop Rh compatibility.

WHAT HAPPENS?

Usually, the blood of a pregnant woman and the fetus do not mix. But under certain circumstances, the blood can mix.

If the blood of an Rh-positive baby mixes with that of an Rh-negative mother, the mother's immune system can make antibodies that can destroy a fetus's red blood cells. This is typically not an issue during a first pregnancy, but if a woman is not treated, these antibodies can put her next baby at risk.

RISKS

- Brain damage due to high levels of bilirubin.
- Fluid buildup and swelling in the baby.
- Impaired mental function, movement, hearing, and speech in baby.
- Hemolytic anemia: depending on the severity, causes jaundice to liver failure.

In the first trimester, the Rh antibodies are typically harmless to the baby, as it takes time for Mom's body to produce the antibodies. It is in the second trimester or later that the greatest risk arises.

TREATMENT

Doctor routinely performs a blood test, at which time they will determine if you have Rh incompatibility. If you have Rh-negative blood, your doctor may order another blood test to check for antibodies.

POSITIVE: If your test comes back positive for antibodies, you are at risk of Rh incompatibility. Your doctor will closely watch to make sure your antibody levels don't get too high.

If incompatibility is severe and the baby is in danger, a special blood transfusion is done before or after birth. This transfusion replaces the baby's blood with fresh blood cells from the mother that have not been damaged by the antibodies.

NEGATIVE: If your test comes back negative, you will be given two shots of a special immune globulin called RhoGAM that prevents the production of antibodies.
1. The first shot at 28 weeks.
2. The second shot within 72 hours after giving birth.
3. You will also receive RhoGAM if you have a miscarriage or ectopic pregnancy.

TREATMENT AFTER BIRTH

Depends on the severity of the condition.

MILD SEVERITY: May be treated with phototherapy using bilirubin lights.
An IV of immune globulin may be used.

HIGH SEVERITY: A transfusion of blood may be done.

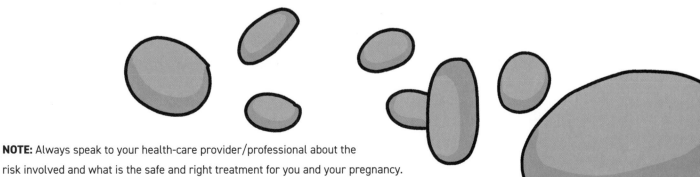

NOTE: Always speak to your health-care provider/professional about the risk involved and what is the safe and right treatment for you and your pregnancy.

FIBROIDS
WHAT TO KNOW WHEN PREGNANT

Fibroids and some of the treatments for them can affect both your fertility and your pregnancy. It's important to talk to your doctor to understand what can be done to have a healthy pregnancy.

WHAT IS IT?

FIBROIDS: A benign tumor/growth of muscle in or on the uterus. They can be large or they can be small; they are usually noncancerous.

Fibroids may increase or decrease in size during pregnancy. Up to 15 percent of women with fibroids experience pain during pregnancy that requires treatment with medication. Talk to your doctor if you experience pain to discuss treatment options.

WHAT CAUSES IT?

The cause of these growths is unknown.

TYPES

SUBSEROSAL FIBROIDS

A fibroid that grows on the surface of the uterus. These are the least likely to cause an issue with getting pregnant, as they are outside the womb.

INTRAMURAL FIBROIDS

A fibroid that grows inside the wall of the uterus. If they become large, they can make it a bit more difficult to get pregnant.

SUBMUCOSAL FIBROIDS

A fibroid that grows inside the womb. These can make it harder to become pregnant, and if you become pregnant, can pose a potential risk to baby.

NOTE: Always speak to your health-care provider/professional about the risk involved and what is the safe and right treatment for you and your pregnancy.

RISKS

Large or numerous fibroids can potentially result in:

- Prolonged periods
- Pressure on the pelvis
- Frequent urination
- Difficult deliveries
- Feeling of fullness

- Excessive bleeding
- Difficulty becoming pregnant
- Difficult bowel movements
- Abnormal placenta
- Requiring a C-section

- Pain
- Premature birth
- Miscarriage
- Breech baby

TREATMENT

There are several procedures used to treat fibroids. You should consult your OB-GYN to understand the procedure and risk to determine what is right for you and your baby.

NOTE: Treatment is typically not done during pregnancy. It important to talk to your doctor about any future plans to become pregnant before undergoing any treatment, as this will affect the treatment options.

MEDICATION:

Medication can be used to manage symptoms and shrink the fibroids. However, taking some medications may prevent you from becoming pregnant. Consult your doctor.

SURGERY (MYOMECTOMY):

A surgical procedure where the fibroid is removed and the uterus reconstructed.

UTERINE FIBROID EMBOLIZATION:

A procedure where the blood supply to the fibroid is blocked, causing the fibroid to shrink; however there are potential pregnancy complications. Consult your doctor.

RADIOFREQUENCY ABLATION:

A surgical procedure where fibroid tissue is heated, causing it to shrink. This is a relatively new procedure, and, therefore, all of the potential side effects may not be known. Consult your doctor.

MRI-GUIDED ULTRASOUND:

The fibroid is destroyed using thermal energy.

PRETERM LABOR
WHAT TO KNOW

WHAT IS IT?

PRETERM LABOR: Labor that occurs before the 37th week of pregnancy, which can result in a premature birth.

CAUSES & RISK FACTORS

The cause for preterm labor is not always known, but there some potential risk factors that can contribute to it:

- Bladder infection
- Smoking or drug abuse
- Diabetes
- Kidney disease
- Lack of prenatal care
- Older than 35
- Pregnancy by IVF
- Exposure to pollutants

- High blood pressure
- Previous preterm births
- Having multiples
- Over or underweight
- Detached placenta
- Younger than 17
- High stress levels

- Vaginal bleeding from uterus
- Infection or inflammation
- Extra amniotic fluid
- Cervix issues
- Poor nutrition
- PPROM
- Injury

NOTE: Always speak to your health-care provider/professional about any health risk or concerns involved and what is the safe and right treatment for you and your pregnancy.

TREATMENT

In some cases, preterm labor stops on its own, but if there is concern that you might have a preterm/premature birth, you may be given several medications to help baby, including:

- Magnesium sulfate: to delay delivery and protect brain.

- Corticosteroids: to help lungs mature.

- Tocolysis: to delay delivery and lessen chance of illness or death of baby.

HOW TO REDUCE RISK

Things to do to try and reduce the risk of early delivery.

- Manage your weight before and during pregnancy.

- Reduce stress.

- Don't smoke, drink alcohol, or abuse drugs.

- Get consistent prenatal care.

- Wait at least 18 months before getting pregnant again.

- Treat and manage health issues.

- Speak to your doctor about vaccinations.

WHEN TO CALL THE DOCTOR

If you are experiencing any of the following symptoms, you should contact your health-care provider:

- Regular and frequent contractions

- Pressure in your pelvis or lower abdomen

- Vaginal bleeding or loss of fluid

- Abdominal cramps without diarrhea

- Constant, low, dull backache

- Water breaking

- Vaginal discharge: watery, bloody, or with mucus

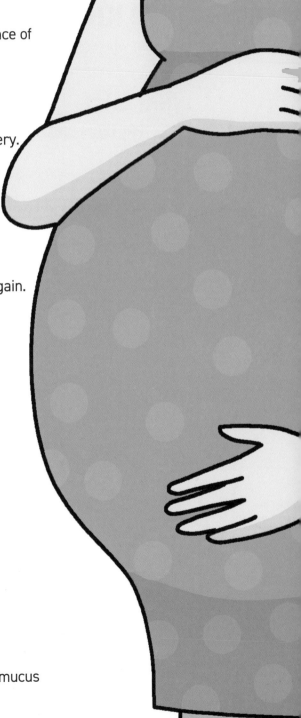

PRETERM BIRTH

WHAT TO KNOW

The who, what, and when of the process of pregnancy.

WHAT IS IT?

PRETERM BIRTH: A birth that takes place before 37 weeks of pregnancy.

TYPES OF PRETERM BIRTHS

Moderate to Late Preterm: Born 32–37 weeks

Very Preterm: Born 28–32 weeks

Extremely Preterm: Born before 28 weeks

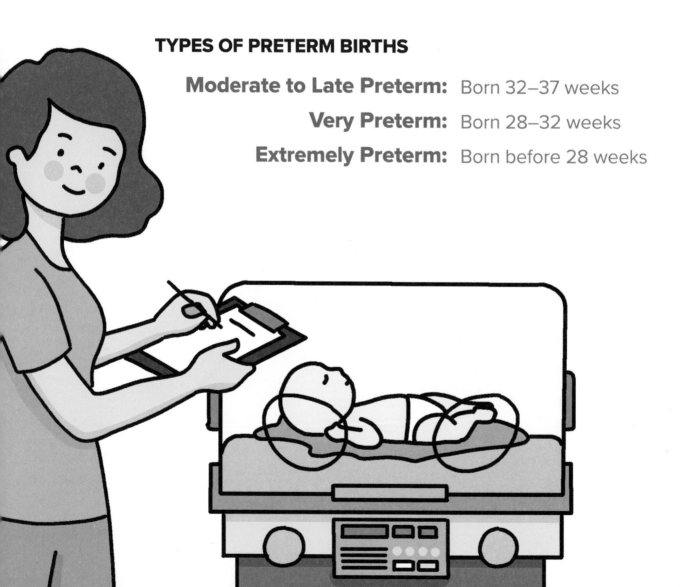

COMPLICATIONS

Having a preemie comes with several potential health issues because the baby has not had time to fully develop. The earlier a baby is born, the greater the potential for complications like these:

- Visual issues
- Hearing issues
- Developmental issues
- Lung disease
- Cerebral palsy
- Bleeding in the brain
- Intestinal issues
- Dental issues

WHEN TO CALL THE DOCTOR

If you are experiencing any of the following symptoms, you should contact your health-care provider:

- Regular and frequent contractions

- Pressure in your pelvis or lower abdomen

- Changes in your vaginal discharge: watery, bloody, or with mucus

- Vaginal bleeding or loss of fluid

- Abdominal cramps without diarrhea

- Constant, low, dull backache

- Water breaking

WHAT HAPPENS AFTER PRETERM BIRTH?

If a woman gives birth early, a team of health professionals will take care of her baby in the Neonatal Intensive Care Unit (NICU), where preterm babies receive specialized care.

Depending on how premature the baby is, it could stay in the NICU for weeks or months.

NOTE: Always speak to your health-care provider/professional about any health risks or concerns involved and what is safe and right treatment for you and your pregnancy.

PROM & PPROM

PRETERM PRELABOR RUPTURE OF MEMBRANES

WHAT IS IT?

PROM

PRELABOR RUPTURE OF MEMBRANES: The breaking of the amniotic sac surrounding baby before actual labor begins, after 37 weeks gestation. This is common and occurs in up to 8 percent of pregnancies.

PPROM

PRETERM PREMATURE RUPTURE OF MEMBRANES: The breaking of the amniotic sac surrounding baby before 37 weeks of pregnancy. This occurs in 2 to 3 percent of pregnancies.

PPROM: CAUSES & RISK FACTORS

- Bladder infection
- Sexually transmitted infection
- Vaginal bleeding
- Low socioeconomic conditions
- Previous preterm birth
- Smoking

RISKS TO BABY

- Premature birth
- Detached placenta
- Infection of placental tissue
- Compressed umbilical cord

RISKS TO MOM

- Postpartum Infection
- Cesarean birth

SYMPTOMS

- Leaking or gush of watery fluid
- Constantly wet underwear

TREATMENT

- Hospitalization for PPROM.

- Monitoring the baby's heart rate, movement, etc.

- Watching for signs of infection, fever, and pain.

- Corticosteroids to help the baby's organs mature.

- Antibiotics to prevent infection.

- Tocolysis to slow preterm labor.

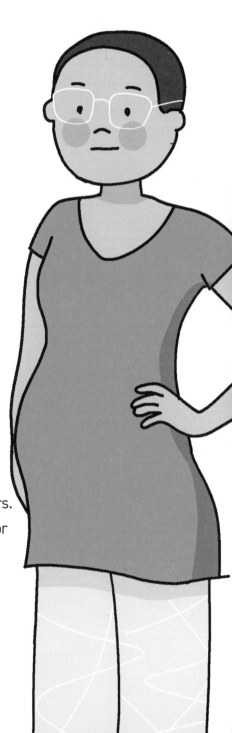

PPROM TREATMENT

In most cases after PPROM, you will be delivered around 34 weeks (if you do not deliver on your own earlier) to balance the risks of prematurity and infection.

PROM TREATMENT

When water breaks before the onset of labor at term (after 37 weeks), about half of women will deliver on their own within 33 hours. The longer the water is broken, the greater the chance of infection for Mom and baby. Therefore, in many cases, labor will be induced or augmented with oxytocin or other medications.

NOTE: Always speak to your health-care provider/professional about the risk involved and what is safe and right for you and your pregnancy.

PREECLAMPSIA
WHAT TO KNOW

WHAT IS IT?

PREECLAMPSIA: A serious blood pressure condition that can develop after 20 weeks of pregnancy or in the postpartum period.

NOTE: Preeclampsia can occur in the postpartum period. In severe cases, it can be life-threatening for women, so if you develop symptoms after delivery, contact your doctor right away.

SYMPTOMS

- High blood pressure
- Loss of vision
- Floaters or spots in the eyes
- Severe pain on the right side
- Protein in urine
- Blurred vision
- Decrease in urine output
- Swelling of legs, hands, & face
- Persistent headache
- Difficulty breathing
- Easy bruising

RISKS & COMPLICATIONS

Left untreated, it is dangerous for both the mother and her baby. It can result in:

- Liver disorder
- Stroke and heart attack
- Cardiovascular disease
- Brain damage
- Detached placenta
- Preterm delivery
- Seizures
- Kidney disease
- High blood pressure

TREATMENT

There is no cure for preeclampsia; the only cure is delivering the baby. To help manage the condition, your doctor might prescribe the use of a low-dose aspirin.

IF 37 WEEKS OR MORE: It might be recommended to deliver baby early.

IF EARLIER THAN 37 WEEKS: The doctor will monitor your pregnancy closely and try to prolong, allowing baby to develop as much as possible.

IF SEVERE PREECLAMPSIA: You may need to stay in the hospital.

CAUSES

It is not completely clear what causes preeclampsia, but there are some common factors in those who have had it:

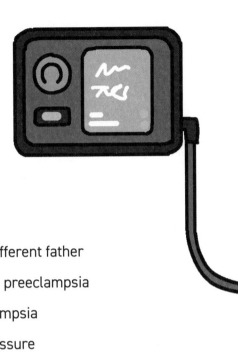

- First pregnancy
- Over 40 years old
- Having multiples
- Diabetes or lupus
- Overweight
- Pregnant via IVF
- Kidney disease
- Blood-clotting disorder
- First pregnancy with a different father
- Previous pregnancy with preeclampsia
- Family history of preeclampsia
- History of high blood pressure
- Less than 2 years or more than 10 years between pregnancies

WHAT TO DO

Some of the symptoms of preeclampsia are common to pregnancy, and many people don't even know that they have it. For this reason, it's important to share all your symptoms with your health-care provider.

Your doctor will likely monitor your condition and perform several tests, including:

- Blood-pressure test.
- Blood test to check the liver and kidney functions.
- Urinalysis to check your protein levels.
- The doctor will also check your baby's vital signs.

NOTE:

Always speak with your health-care provider, and let them know about any symptoms so they can monitor them and determine the right course of action.

HIGH BLOOD PRESSURE

GETTING STARTED

High blood pressure can manifest itself in several ways during pregnancy.

WHAT IS IT?

HIGH BLOOD PRESSURE: Also called hypertension, it occurs when the force of the blood against the artery walls is too high. Over time, if untreated, it can cause other health conditions, such as heart disease and stroke.

HIGH BLOOD PRESSURE & PREGNANCY

During pregnancy, there are several potential high-blood-pressure disorders:

PREECLAMPSIA: A dangerous blood pressure condition (see previous page).

GESTATIONAL HYPERTENSION: This type begins after 20 weeks; there are no symptoms of preeclampsia.

CHRONIC HYPERTENSION: High blood pressure that was present before pregnancy or occurs before 20 weeks of pregnancy.

CHRONIC HYPERTENSION WITH SUPERIMPOSED PREECLAMPSIA: Happens in women who had chronic high blood pressure before becoming pregnant and have developed worsening high blood pressure along with protein in their urine or other complications during pregnancy.

RISKS

High blood pressure during pregnancy can prevent the placenta from receiving enough blood, which can result in:

- Seizures in Mom
- Stroke
- Liver problems
- Blood clots
- Preterm delivery
- Cesarean
- Placenta detaching
- Kidney problems

If you have high blood pressure prior to 20 weeks, or other risk factors for preeclampsia, talk to your doctor about ways to prevent preeclampsia. In some cases, baby aspirin may be recommended.

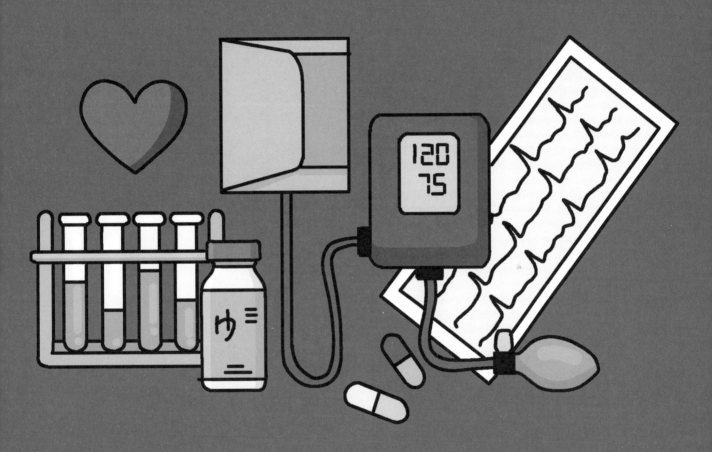

NOTE: Always speak to your health-care provider/professional about the risk involved and what is the safe and right treatment for you and your pregnancy.

CERVICAL INSUFFICIENCY
WHAT IS IT?

WHAT IS IT?

CERVICAL INSUFFICIENCY: Also called cervical incompetence. The cervix is the tissue that connects the vagina and the uterus. Sometimes the cervix opens and thins prematurely during the second trimester. When it does, it is called cervical insufficiency.

QUICK TIP

The use of monofilament/non-braided sutures has been found to be associated with lower risk of infection. Consult your doctor.

WOMEN AT RISK

Women are at a greater risk of cervical insufficiency if they:

- Had cervical trauma.
- Had a cervical biopsy.
- Are in the second trimester.
- Had an earlier operation on the cervix.
- Have a history of late-term miscarriage.

TREATMENT

After checking your baby's health and confirming that you do not have any infection, an emergency cerclage might be performed.

CERCLAGE: A procedure to temporarily stitch the cervix closed with a band of thread, essentially helping to keep the cervix closed or from opening further.
The success rate is fairly high.

RISKS:
- Infection of stitched area
- Water breaking
- Vaginal bleeding
- Premature contractions
- Preterm delivery or miscarriage
- Tearing of the cervix

The cerclage typically will stay in place until you reach full-term and are ready for delivery, at which time it is removed.

CERVICAL INSUFFICIENCY

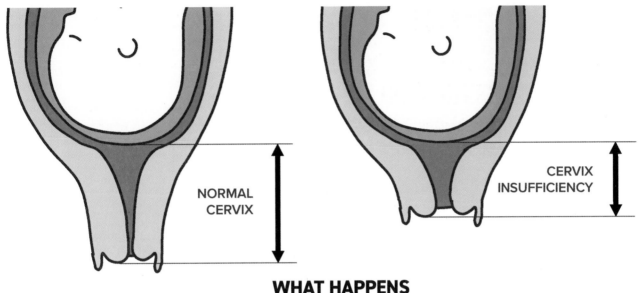

NORMAL CERVIX

CERVIX INSUFFICIENCY

WHAT HAPPENS
The cervix thins/shortens and opens

TYPES OF CERCLAGE

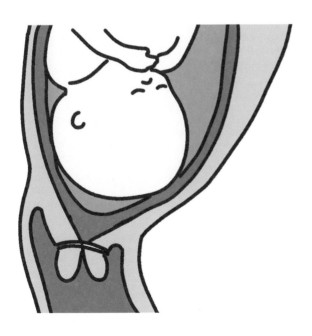

THREE TYPES OF CERCLAGE

MCDONALD CERCLAGE: The most common, using a band of suture at the upper part of the cervix.

SHIRODKAR CERCLAGE: Sutures are placed higher on the cervix than a McDonald cerclage and require a more involved surgical dissection.

ABDOMINAL CERCLAGE: A band is placed at the very top, outside of the cervix and inside the abdomen. This is a permanent procedure and requires a C-section for delivery.

NOTE: Always speak to your health-care provider/professional about the risk involved and what is safe and right for you and your pregnancy.

THYROID DISEASE

GETTING STARTED

The thyroid makes hormones that help regulate how your body works; too little or too much can cause problems during pregnancy.

WHAT IS IT?

THE THYROID: The thyroid is a gland that produces hormones that regulate how your body uses energy; it affects most organs in your body and your heart.

THYROID DISEASE: A disorder that affects the gland's production of hormones.

HYPERTHYROIDISM: The production of **too much** hormone—meaning that the thyroid is overactive.

HYPOTHYROIDISM: The production of **too little** hormone—meaning that the thyroid is underactive.

THE THYROID & PREGNANCY

Thyroid hormones play an essential role in the development of a baby's brain and nervous system. During the first several months (until around week 20, when theirs start to work), your baby depends on your thyroid.

RISK OF THYROID CONDITION

You are at a higher risk of developing the condition if:

- You currently have a thyroid condition.

- You have had a thyroid condition.

- You have an autoimmune disorder or family history of one.

- You have type 1 diabetes.

- You have had radiation treatment for hyperthyroidism.

HYPERTHYROIDISM (OVERACTIVE):

This thyroid condition during pregnancy is commonly caused by Graves' disease (an autoimmune disease).

Complications of hyperthyroidism for Mom:

- Severe form of morning sickness, with excessive vomiting and nausea
- Preeclampsia
- Pulmonary hypertension
- The placenta detaching from the uterus
- Heart failure

Complications of hyperthyroidism for baby:

- Premature birth
- Goiter
- Low birth weight
- Thyroid problems
- Miscarriage or stillbirth

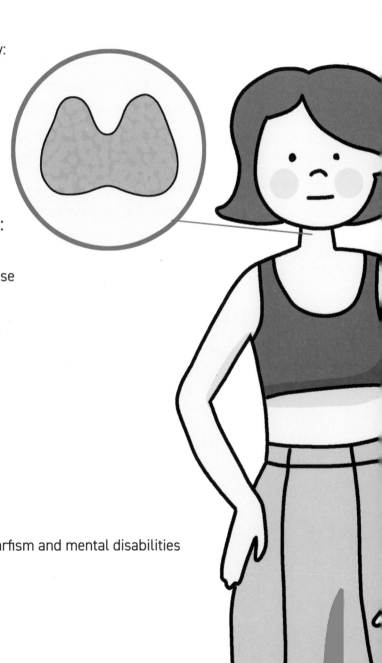

HYPOTHYROIDISM (UNDERACTIVE):

This thyroid condition during pregnancy is commonly caused by Hashimoto's disease (an autoimmune disorder).

Complications of hypothyroidism for Mom:

- Anemia
- Gestational hypertension
- Preeclampsia
- Heavy bleeding postpartum
- Myxedema: coma or death
- Heart failure

Complications of hypothyroidism for baby:

- Infantile myxedema: causing dwarfism and mental disabilities
- Low birth weight
- Thyroid problems
- Miscarriage or stillbirth

GESTATIONAL DIABETES

GETTING STARTED

What you need to know about gestational diabetes.

QUICK TIP

Many women with gestational diabetes will develop type 2 diabetes after pregnancy, so it is important to speak with your doctor to help prevent it.

WHAT IS IT?

GESTATIONAL DIABETES: A type of diabetes (high blood sugar) that can affect moms-to-be when they are pregnant. It usually happens in the later part of pregnancy.

WHAT CAUSES IT?

It happens when the body becomes resistant to insulin in pregnancy, resulting in blood sugar levels that are too high. The changes of pregnancy affect the body's cells' ability to use insulin effectively, which raises mom's blood sugar levels.

Your blood sugar level usually returns to normal after baby is born; however:

50% of women who have gestational diabetes may potentially develop type 2 diabetes.

You can lower this risk of developing type 2 diabetes by:

- Having a healthy body weight before pregnancy.
- Reaching a healthy body weight after pregnancy.
- Having your blood sugar levels tested 6 to 12 weeks after delivery and every one to three years to track and maintain those levels.
- Exercising regularly.

RISKS TO BABY

Untreated high blood sugar level in mom can cause baby to:

- Be born large (9 lbs. or more).
- Have low blood sugar levels.
- Develop type 2 diabetes later in life.

- Be born premature.
- Be stillborn.
- Have respiratory related complications.

TIPS FOR MANAGING DIABETES

MONITOR SUGAR LEVELS

Make sure you monitor your blood sugar levels to stay in a healthy range. Follow any medication regimen your doctor prescribes.

EAT HEALTHILY

Eat a healthy diet that is high in fiber, grains, fruits, and vegetables and that is low in calories and fat. Also, control portion size. Consult a nutritionist about creating a healthy meal plan to meet your specific pregnancy needs.

EXERCISE

Stay active with regular, moderate-level exercise, like walking. Speak to your doctor about what the best exercise is for you and your pregnancy.

MONITOR BABY

Go to your prenatal appointment so that your health-care provider can monitor your baby's development.

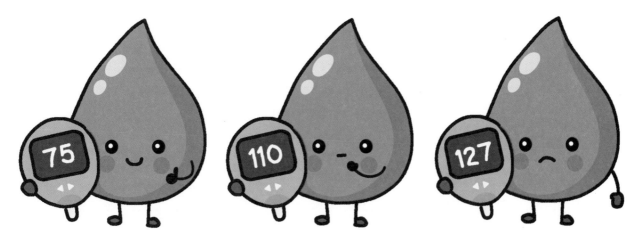

PLACENTA ISSUES

The placenta plays a critical role in the development of your baby, so it is important for you to be on the lookout for some conditions of concern. Here is what you need to know.

THE PLACENTA

An organ that develops in the uterus during pregnancy, that is the bridge between mother and baby. It provides oxygen and nutrients to the baby and removes waste products from its blood. The placenta is attached to the uterus, and the umbilical cord attaches to the baby.

PLACENTA ISSUES

PLACENTAL ABRUPTION: When the placenta detaches—partially or completely—from the wall of the uterus before delivery. This can reduce the amount of oxygen and nutrients that the baby gets and cause heavy bleeding.

PLACENTAL PREVIA: A condition where the placenta either partially or completely covers the opening of the uterus. Typically happening early in pregnancy, it may correct itself as the uterus grows with the baby, pulling away from the opening. Placenta previa can cause heavy bleeding during pregnancy or delivery; in the latter case, if placenta previa does not resolve, a C-section is required.

PLACENTA ACCRETA: When the placenta grows too deeply into the wall of the uterus. Typically, the placenta detaches after your baby is born and is delivered, but with placenta accreta, all or part of the placenta remains attached. This can cause intense bleeding. A C-section may be needed to remove the placenta, and depending on the depth of attachment, the uterus might need to be removed too.

RETAINED PLACENTA: When the placenta does not deliver within 30 minutes of childbirth, it's called a retained placenta. This can cause infection and dangerous blood loss.

3 TYPES OF PLACENTA PREVIA

NORMAL PLACENTA LOCATION

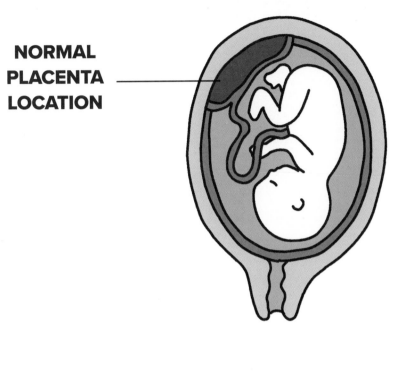

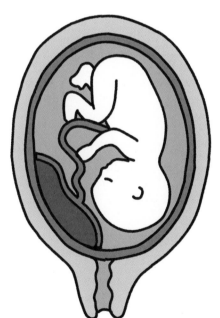

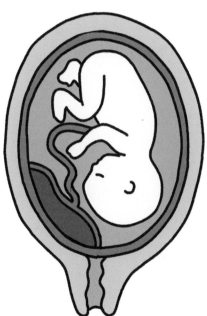

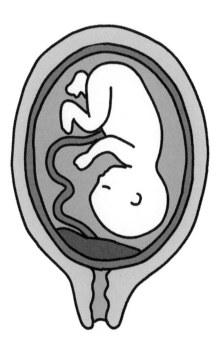

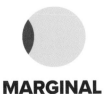

MARGINAL

PARTIAL

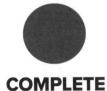

COMPLETE

TOXOPLASMOSIS
BAD KITTY

TOXOPLASMOSIS

This infection is caused by a parasite (toxoplasma gondii), which is found in cat feces as well as in contaminated foods.

HOW YOU GET IT

People can become accidentally infected by ingesting the microscopic eggs of the parasite either:

- From cleaning a cat's litter box or anything infected by it.
- Eating or drinking any infected meat, fish, water, fruits, or vegetables.

COMPLICATIONS

Most people's immune systems fight off the infection, but toxoplasmosis can cause serious health issues for pregnant moms and their babies, including:

- Preterm birth
- Stillbirth
- Miscarriage

Baby could experience:

- Liver and spleen damage
- Brain damage
- Eye inflammation & infections
- Jaundice
- Seizures
- Swollen lymph nodes
- Low birth weight
- Rash or bruising
- Cerebral palsy

TREATMENT IF INFECTED

During pregnancy:

- You and your baby will be monitored during pregnancy and after birth.
- You will get an antibiotic treatment to reduce the chance your baby gets infected.

Baby shows signs of infection after birth:

- Baby may be treated with antibiotics for their first year or longer.

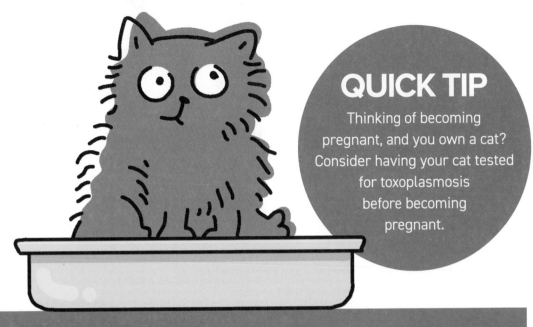

QUICK TIP

Thinking of becoming pregnant, and you own a cat? Consider having your cat tested for toxoplasmosis before becoming pregnant.

TIPS TO PREVENT TOXOPLASMOSIS

NO RAW MEAT

Make sure that meats, lamb, pork, venison, and beef are cooked thoroughly.

NO RAW SEAFOOD

Don't eat raw, undercooked shellfish or seafood; don't drink raw, unpasteurized milk.

KIDS' SANDBOX

Cover kids' sandboxes so cats don't use them as a litter box.

WASH

Be sure to wash fruits, vegetables, utensils, surfaces, cutting boards, and your hands after handling food products.

WEAR GLOVES

Avoid gardening or wear gloves in areas a cat might have soiled; wash hands thoroughly.

KITTY LITTER

Ask someone to change the litter box, or wear gloves if you do it; it's best to change it daily.

KEEP CATS INSIDE

To prevent your cats from getting contaminated, keep them inside.

STRAY CATS

Don't touch stray cats or kittens.

CAT FOOD

Feed cats canned or commercial food; don't feed your pet raw or undercooked meats.

STDS
PROTECTING YOU AND BABY

When you are pregnant, STDs can have a serious effect on you and your baby. Here is what you need to know about them.

STDS (SEXUALLY TRANSMITTED DISEASES)

Infections that are spread by having sex with someone who is infected with an STD.

HOW YOU GET IT

STDs are spread through sex involving the mouth, anus, or vagina with someone who has an STD.

WHAT ARE THEY?

STDs include:

- Chlamydia
- Hepatitis B
- Syphilis
- Genital herpes
- HIV/AIDS
- Trichomonas vaginalis
- Gonorrhea
- Gential warts (HPV)

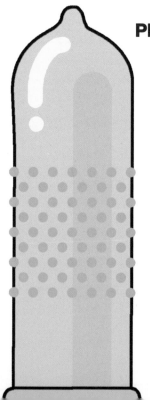

PREVENTION

- Not having sex is the only sure way to prevent STDs.
- Use a condom every time you have sex.
- Limit the number of sex partners.
- Practice monogamy with a partner who has tested negative for any STD.
- Don't use alcohol or drugs before having sex; you might be less likely to practice safe sex if you are high.
- Learn about STDs and the symptoms.

NOTE: Always speak to your health-care provider/professional about the risk involved and what is safe and right for you and your pregnancy.

STD	RISK TO MOM	BABY RISK	TREATMENT
CHLAMYDIA	Vaginal discharge, burning with urination, infertility due to damage to the fallopian tubes.	Severe eye infection, pneumonia, and increased risk of miscarriage.	Mothers are treated with antibiotics; babies are given antibiotic eye ointment at birth.
HERPES	Relatively safe until she gets ready to deliver. Blisters on the genitals, rectum, or mouth.	Can infect the baby during delivery; can damage eyes and nervous system.	Antiviral meds given; C-section is performed if Mom has an active lesion at delivery.
GONORRHEA	Can cause mouth sores, fever, and blood stream infection; vaginal discharge and burning when urinating.	Babies born while Mom has active infection can cause eye infection, blindness, joint or blood infection.	Mothers are treated with antibiotics; babies are given antibiotic eye ointment at birth.
HEPATITIS B	Fatigue, poor appetite, jaundice, liver infection leading to cirrhosis or liver cancer.	Fatigue, poor appetite, jaundice, liver infection leading to cirrhosis or liver cancer.	Newborns get an injection of antibodies and a vaccine to prevent infection.
HIV / AIDS	Virus leads to immunocompromised opportunistic infections and AIDS.	Medications have reduced transmission; if passed on to baby they could develop HIV.	Maintaining a low or negative viral load on antiviral meds; treating infants at delivery can help prevent infection.
SYPHILIS	Sores on the genitals, rectum, or mouth. In late stages, can affect the brain and nervous system.	Easily passed on to an unborn baby, and likely to cause fatal infections. Causes development issues of eyes, ears, skin, heart, and bones.	Antibiotics given to reduce risk of transmission.
TRICHOMONAS VAGINALIS	Foul-smelling vaginal discharge, pain with urination, itching or burning of the genitals.	Untreated can cause premature birth and low birth weight.	Treated with antibiotics.
HPV GENITAL WARTS	Some strains of HPV are associated with cancer as well.	HPV may be passed from mother to infant, but it is a rare occurrence.	Treatment delayed until after delivery, unless warts are very large.

MISCARRIAGE

Unfortunately, miscarriages are relatively common: 10 to 20 percent of all pregnancies end in a miscarriage, which usually happens in the first trimester.

QUICK TIP

A significant number of women who have had a miscarriage subsequently go on to have normal pregnancies and births.

WHAT IS IT?

MISCARRIAGE: The loss of baby before 20 weeks of pregnancy.

CAUSES

The exact causes of a miscarriage can be difficult to determine. Miscarriages often happen when the fetus is not developing normally, with potential causes including:

- Genetic abnormality of the embryo or fetus

- Abnormal chromosomes or genes

- Certain illnesses, like diabetes, hormonal issues, or thyroid disease

- Serious infection

- A major injury

- Abnormalities of the uterus (such as fibroids or a uterine septum)

- A previous miscarriage

TYPES OF MISCARRIAGES

THREATENED MISCARRIAGE: There is bleeding and mild cramps, but the cervix stays closed. In half of these occurrences, the bleeding stops and the pregnancy proceeds normally. Unfortunately, the other half may result in loss of the pregnancy.

INEVITABLE MISCARRIAGE: Occurs when there is bleeding and the cervix opens—a miscarriage is likely.

INCOMPLETE MISCARRIAGE: Some of the pregnancy tissue is expelled, but some remains in the uterus. This requires a procedure to remove the remaining tissue.

COMPLETE MISCARRIAGE: All the pregnancy tissue is expelled from the uterus.

MISSED MISCARRIAGE: When the embryo is no longer viable, but there is no bleeding or other signs of miscarriage.

RISK FACTORS

- Older than 35
- Diabetes
- Smoking
- Under- or overweight
- Exposure to chemicals
- History of miscarriages
- Uterine or cervical issues
- Alcohol or drug abuse
- After a CVS or amniocentesis
- Autoimmune disorder

TREATMENT

Your doctor may first run some tests, including:

- A pelvic exam
- Ultrasound test
- Blood test
- Tissue test
- Uterus examination
- Genetic testing

Treatment may include medication and a procedure to remove any pregnancy tissue that was not expelled by the body.

It may take four to six weeks for the body to recover from a miscarriage.

EMOTIONALLY: Having a miscarriage is a very personal experience that can result in a range of emotions from sadness to guilt to grief. These reactions are completely normal. It can take some time to recover emotionally from a miscarriage. Refer to the section on dealing with loss.

NOTE: Always speak to your health-care provider/professional about the risk involved and what is safe and right for you and your pregnancy.

STILLBIRTH

Stillbirths are a sad reality for many families and can take a deep emotional toll on them.

WHAT IS IT?

STILLBIRTH: The loss of a baby after 20 weeks of pregnancy or during delivery.

TYPES OF STILLBIRTHS

EARLY STILLBIRTH: Loss occurring between 20 and 27 weeks.

LATE STILLBIRTH: Loss occurring between 28 and 36 weeks.

TERM STILLBIRTH: Loss occurring at 37 or more weeks.

CAUSES & RISK FACTORS

The exact causes of stillbirths are often unknown, but some potential causes are:

- Congenital anomalies
- Premature birth
- Some impairment of fetal growth
- Medical conditions: diabetes, renal disease, heart conditions, or preeclampsia
- Issues with the placenta or umbilical cord

Other things that might increase the risk of having a stillbirth:

- Domestic violence
- Sleeping on your back
- Moms 35 years or older
- Moms who smoke during pregnancy
- Moms who have diabetes or are overweight
- Having multiples
- Previous lost pregnancies
- Poor prenatal care

PREVENTION

Even though the exact cause of a stillbirth is often unknown, there are things you can do that may lower your risk of having one; among them:

HEALTHY HABITS: Eating healthy and taking your prenatal vitamins.

AVOIDING ALCOHOL: Not drinking alcohol, smoking, or taking drugs.

PRENATAL APPOINTMENTS: Going to your prenatal appointments and screenings.

MANAGE HEALTH CONDITIONS: Treat high blood pressure, diabetes, and other issues.

SLEEPING POSITION: Sleep on your left side during the third trimester.

DELIVERY

In most cases, your health-care provider will recommend that you deliver vaginally.

- Physical recovery is faster than a C-section.
- There is less risk of infection and bleeding.
- You will have more time to process events while your body prepares for labor.
- C-section results in increased risks of placental abnormalities with next pregnancies.

DIAGNOSIS

Your doctor may examine you and run some tests to discover the cause:

- Pelvic exam
- Ultrasound test
- Blood test
- Genetic testing
- Examination of the umbilical cord
- Examination of the placenta
- Tests for infection

The doctor may also, with your consent, perform an autopsy.

RECOVERY

It may take a few weeks or a month for the body to recover from a stillbirth; however, emotionally it is a traumatic experience, and it is normal to experience a range of emotions, from sadness and guilt to grief. It will take time to recover emotionally from a stillbirth; see the chapter on dealing with loss.

NOTE: Always speak to your health-care provider/professional about the risk involved and what is safe and right for you and your pregnancy.

AMNIOCENTESIS
BEING READY FOR BABY MENTALLY

The who, what, and when of the process of pregnancy.

WHAT IS IT?

AMNIOCENTESIS: A test used to diagnose chromosomal disorders and neural tube defects. It involves taking a small sample of the amniotic fluid that surrounds the fetus.

WHY DO IT?

The test is generally offered at: 15 to 20 weeks for women who are at increased risk of chromosomal abnormalities.

Includes women:

- Over 35 years of age.
- Who have tested positive during prenatal screening.
- With a history or previous pregnancy with genetic issues.
- Who had an abnormal ultrasound finding.

HOW IS IT DONE?

The procedure involves collecting a small amount of amniotic fluid. A needle, guided by an ultrasound, is inserted through the abdomen into the amniotic sac. The fluid collected contains enzymes, proteins, hormones, and other substances. It is tested for protein levels, which are an indicator of certain defects. Cells in the fluid are also tested for chromosomal disorders and genetic problems.

COMPLICATIONS

· Cramping	· Infection	· Miscarriage
· Preterm labor	· Bleeding	· Leakage of amniotic fluid

NOTE: Always speak to your health-care provider/professional about the risk involved and what is safe and right for you and your pregnancy.

AMNIOCENTESIS PROCESS

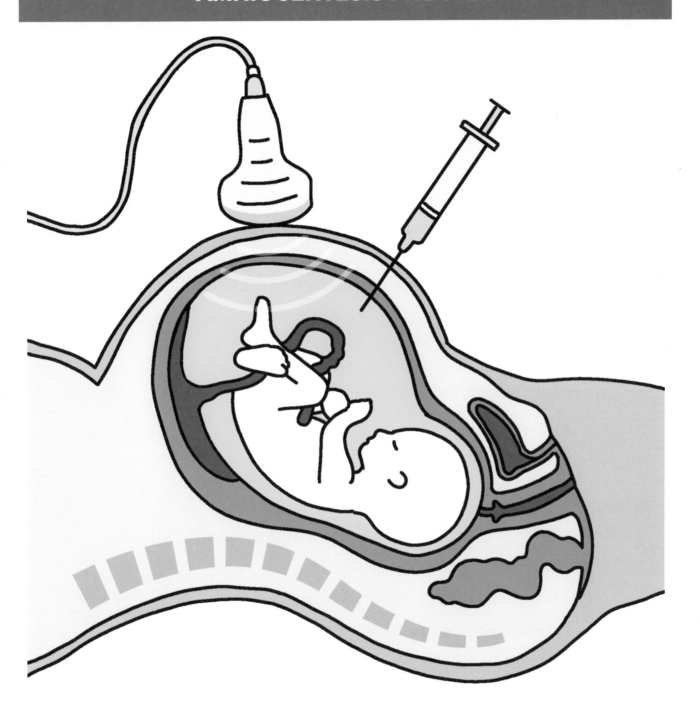

THINGS TESTED FOR

- Muscular dystrophy
- RH disease
- Neural tube defects
- Chromosomal abnormalities
- Lung maturity
- Genetic disorders

BIRTH DEFECTS
UNDERSTANDING THE RISK

Unfortunately, birth defects are more common than you might think, and it's important to understand what they are and how you can improve your chances of your baby not having one.

WHAT IS IT?

BIRTH DEFECT: A developmental issue that affects various parts of the body, including how the body looks, or works, or both. Birth defects can range from mild to severe and can happen at any stage of pregnancy. Most occur in the first three months of pregnancy, when the organs are forming.

CAUSES

It is difficult to know the cause of most birth defects. Many defects are the result of a combination of factors, including:

- Genetics
- Infections
- Chromosomal problems
- Lack of nutrients
- Toxic exposure
- Certain medications

RISKS

Things that increase the chances of having a baby with a birth defect:

- Smoking, alcohol, or drug abuse
- Certain medical conditions, like obesity and diabetes
- Certain medications, like isotretinoin
- Family history of birth defects
- Certain infections during pregnancy
- Fever greater than 101°F or an elevated body temperature
- Age 35 years or older

NOTE: Always speak to your health-care provider/professional about the risk involved and what is safe and right for you and your pregnancy.

PREVENTION

Things you can do to increase your chances of having a healthy baby:

PRENATAL CARE: Be sure to attend all your prenatal care appointments to ensure you and your baby are getting good care.

FOLIC ACID: Get 400 micrograms of folic acid every day, and make sure you take your prenatal vitamins. Take at least one month before getting pregnant.

ALCOHOL: Don't drink alcohol.

SMOKING: Don't smoke.

MEDICATIONS: Be sure to speak with your health-care provider about any medications you are taking, including prescriptions, over-the-counter medication, and herbal supplements.

MANAGE FEVERS: If you become sick with a fever of 101°F or greater, speak to your doctor right away so it can be appropriately managed.

KEEP COOL: Avoid hot tubs, saunas, or any environment that is overly hot.

MEDICAL CONDITIONS: Be sure to manage any preexisting medical conditions with your health-care provider.

MANAGE YOUR WEIGHT: Manage your weight; obesity is a risk factor.

VACCINATIONS: Speak to your health-care provider to make sure you are up to date on any needed vaccinations.

DIAGNOSIS

Diagnosing birth defects can be done through:

- Prenatal testing
- Newborn screening

Be kind
to your
mind.

MENTAL HEALTH

You may have many feelings and emotions throughout pregnancy—some good, some bad.

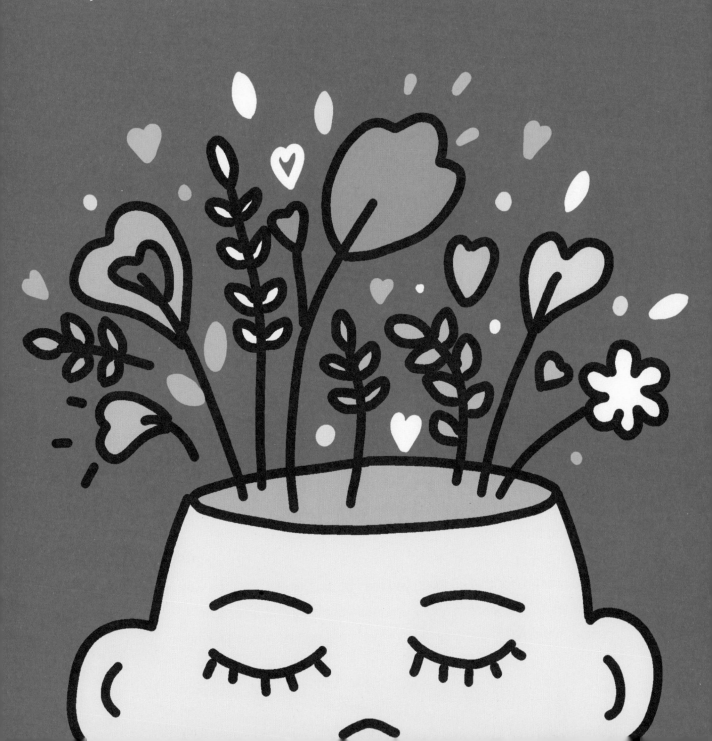

PREPARING FOR BABY

CHANGE; IT'S ABOUT TO BE DELIVERED TOO!

Having a baby is one of the biggest changes in life, and being prepared mentally for those changes can make the transition much smoother.

OVERVIEW

It can't be overstated that having a baby brings major changes in your life—many expected and many you didn't see coming. Getting mentally prepared for these changes is a good idea. It won't stop you from having that, "OMG, I had no idea moment!" that all parents have, but at least it will help reduce a few of those head snaps.

TIPS FOR PREPARING FOR BABY

WHO COMES FIRST?

First and foremost, the change you will be experiencing is the realization that you are no longer the center of your universe. It's important to understand that once your baby arrives, it will be the priority. We all kind of know this, but at some point, it really sinks in—painfully at times. Babies demand attention, and everything tends to revolve around them and their needs.

If you prepare for this up front, you may be able to organize the way you structure your activities so that you are able to maintain some kind of a personal life. Being able to get some "me time" is good, because, trust me, it will be sorely lacking.

GET ORGANIZED

Having a baby, especially your first, comes with a host of changes to your life. It is hard to quite grasp how different life becomes once your baby arrives. This uncertainty can create anxiety and stress. Getting organized before baby arrives can help ease those feelings.

Spend time understanding your finances, and how you and your partner will share roles and responsibilities—who will be doing what. Speak to your employer and understand how that work-life balance will be affected.

YOU GOT THIS

Most parents worry whether they have what it takes to care for a baby. We are here to tell you that you do! Will you make mistakes? Yes, everyone does, but your baby is not looking for perfect parents (honestly, they don't exist). What your baby needs is loving, caring, and nurturing parents.

BE NICE!

Having a baby can be stressful and at times overwhelming. You will be tired, you will be anxious, and your patience will be tested, repeatedly. Remember you and your partner are in this together, so it is important to try to be gentle with each other. Talk about this up front so that when those trying moments arise, you know how to speak to each other.

SUPPORT

Before baby shows up, it is a wise idea to try and get your support system in place. Don't assume; find out if your family or friends might be a source of support.

GOT KIDS?

Begin preparing the rest of the family for the new baby. Some kids are thrilled to have a new sibling, but there can also be fear and jealousy. It helps to set aside time and pay attention to your kids. Help them feel part of the pregnancy, for example, by picking out baby items and helping prepare the space.

I'M PREGNANT
HOORAY! hooray?

Having a baby sometimes brings a mix of emotions: overwhelming joy, just not feeling it, or even negative thoughts.

OVERVIEW

OK, let's be honest, not everyone is completely thrilled that they are having a baby. I assume it's far more common than one might think. You thought you were done having kids, or are on birth control, and then, hello, you have a little surprise.

This can be a very stressful and scary situation; what to do now? For many people, this is an extremely complicated place to be.

These mixed feelings can even be felt by parents who want to have a baby. The realization that, "Yes, I'm going to be a mom or a dad," can bring up feelings of anxiety about whether or not you can actually do it.

DITCH THE GUILT

First, let me say, you are not a bad person for having the feelings you have. They are your feelings, and they are valid and OK! It doesn't make you a bad mom or dad to be experiencing them, and, honestly, no one should be judging how you FEEL. Having a baby is a big deal—it affects almost all aspects of your life; so, of course, you are going to have a range of feelings.

We really need to stop discounting the negative ones we experience because it is culturally uncomfortable. It's dishonest to ourselves and doesn't help anyone to pretend that they don't exist. Instead, I believe it would be better to stop focusing on what we're not feeling and examine what we are. Understanding your worries and anxiety is important.

TALK IT OUT

Confiding in someone—your partner, a good friend, family member, other parents, or a health-care provider you trust—can help you understand and address your fears, concerns, and anxieties.

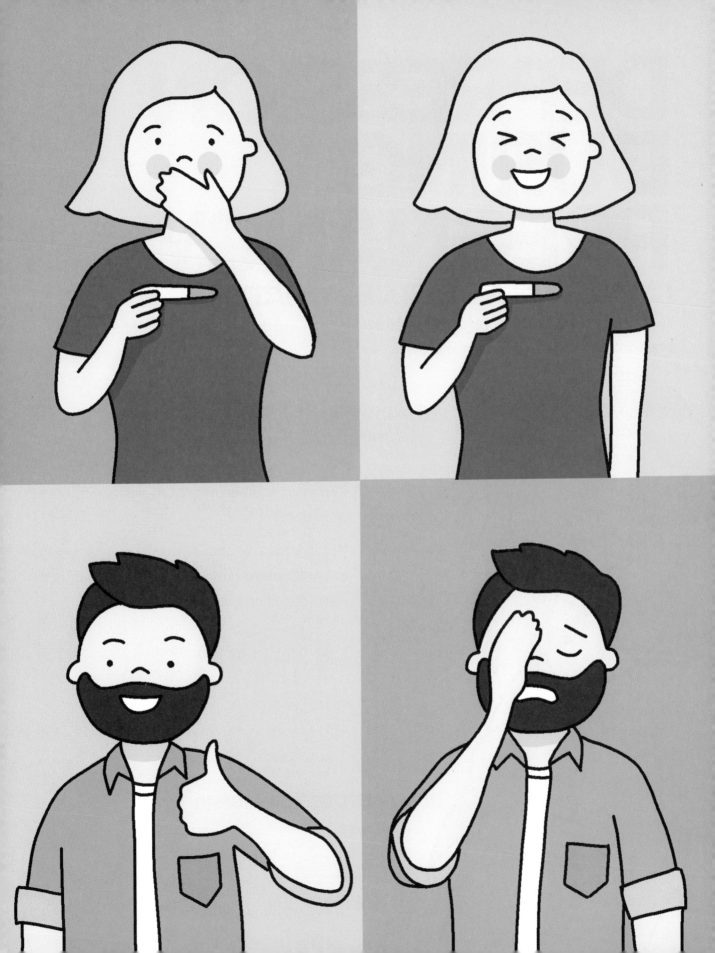

DEPRESSION DURING PREGNANCY

I'M FEELING A BIT BLUE—WHAT'S UP?

We have all heard about depression after birth, but it can and does happen even while you are pregnant. Here is what you need to know.

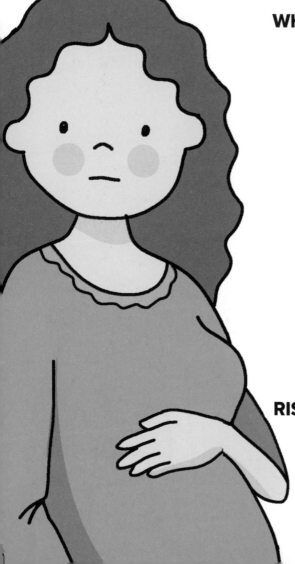

WHAT IS IT?

DEPRESSION: A mood disorder involving persistent feelings of sadness, hopelessness, and loss of interest in activities, which can significantly impair one's daily life.

It occurs twice as often in women as in men. It can go unrecognized during pregnancy, as some of the symptoms of pregnancy can be similar.

AROUND

1 in 10

pregnant women experience
depression during pregnancy

ACCORDING TO THE (ACOG.)

RISK FACTORS & TRIGGERS

- Anxiety
- Stress
- Domestic violence
- Relationship issues
- History of depression
- Lack of support
- Unplanned pregnancy
- Depression runs in family

CAUSES

It is not known for sure what causes depression, but potentially it may be a combination of emotional, physical, and environmental factors. Strong contributors are hormones and genetics.

SYMPTOMS

- Persistent sadness
- Too much or too little sleep
- Suicidal thoughts
- Frequent crying

- Difficulty concentrating
- Loss of interest in daily activities
- Change in eating habits
- Irritability and agitation

- Anxiety
- Hopelessness
- Alcohol Consumption
- Fatigue or low energy

Depression is an illness, not a choice. It's not your fault; it's a medical condition.

TREATMENT

Depression during pregnancy can be treated and managed. If you feel you are experiencing depression, speak to your health-care provider, who may recommend one or a combination of the following:

- Support groups
- Anti-depressants

- Private counseling
- Light therapy

NATURAL TREATMENTS:

- Exercise
- Healthy diet
- Acupuncture
- Spending time with others

- Sleep the right amount
- Less caffeine and sugars
- Omega-3 fatty acids

NOTE: If you think you are experiencing depression, talk to your health-care provider. Only a qualified health-care provider can diagnose depression.

If you have thoughts of hurting yourself or baby, call 911 or the National Suicide Prevention Lifeline: **1-800-273-8255, SMS 988** or text

Crisis line: **Text HELLO to 741741.**

POSTPARTUM DEPRESSION

WHAT YOU NEED TO KNOW

The birth of your baby is supposed to be one of the happiest times in your life, so why do you feel so miserable?

TYPES OF CHILDBIRTH DEPRESSION

There are three kinds of depression a new mother might experience after the birth of her baby. They may be caused by the rapid change in hormone levels that occur after birth.

1. POSTPARTUM BLUES OR BABY BLUES

A common, mild form of after-birth depression beginning within two to three days after delivery and lasting up to two weeks.

2. POSTPARTUM DEPRESSION

A more severe form of depression—the symptoms last longer (more than two weeks) and are more severe.

3. POSTPARTUM PSYCHOSIS

This is a rare but serious condition.

BABY BLUES SYMPTOMS

- Mood swings
- Irritability
- Reduced concentration
- Anxiety
- Feeling overwhelmed
- Changes in appetite
- Feeling blue or sad
- Crying
- Sleeping issues

POSTPARTUM DEPRESSION SYMPTOMS

- Insomnia
- Lack of bonding with baby
- Intense mood swings
- Suicidal thoughts
- Changes in appetite
- Feeling withdrawn
- Frequent crying
- Thoughts of harming baby
- Intense irritability and anger
- Feeling sad and overwhelmed
- Panic attacks

POSTPARTUM PSYCHOSIS SYMPTOMS

- Confusion and disorientation
- Hallucinations and delusions
- Excessive energy and agitation
- Attempts to harm yourself or your baby
- Obsessive thoughts about your baby
- Sleep disturbances
- Paranoia

WHAT TO KNOW & HOW TO TREAT IT

THE BABY BLUES: Feeling sad and/or empty is very common, and this usually goes away in two weeks. Rest when you can, and get help from friends and family.

POSTPARTUM DEPRESSION is a serious condition and needs to be treated. The common treatments for postpartum depression are:

Therapy: Working with a therapist, psychologist, or social worker to learn strategies to understand and manage your depression.

Medication: An antidepressant medication may be prescribed to improve your mood and emotions.

POSTPARTUM PSYCHOSIS is a medical emergency. Call 911 and seek treatment immediately. Treatments during a psychotic episode include medications to reduce depression, stabilize moods, and reduce psychosis.

WHEN TO CALL THE DOCTOR

It's important to call your doctor as soon as possible if the signs and symptoms of depression have any of these features:

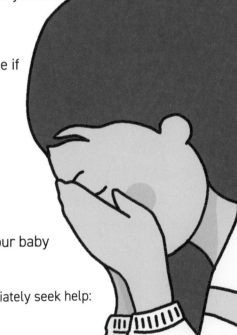

- Don't fade after two weeks
- Get worse
- Make it hard for you to care for your baby
- Make it hard to complete everyday tasks
- Include thoughts of harming yourself or your baby

WARNING

If you have any thoughts of harming yourself or your baby, immediately seek help:

- Contact your primary-care provider.
- Call a mental-health professional.
- Call the National Suicide Prevention Lifeline at **1-800-273-8255.**
- Reach out to a close friend or loved one.

C-SECTION GUILT

You may experience a range of emotions after having a C-section. While some women feel happy about having a C-section, and may even elect to have one, others feel depressed, sad, and ashamed—why?

WHAT IS IT?

C-SECTION GUILT: Some moms blame themselves for not having had their baby the traditional or "natural" way, meaning a vaginal delivery.

GUILT

This type of guilt is triggered by several questions or thoughts.

- If giving birth is "natural," why couldn't I do it?
- I planned for the birth to be one way; why did I end up having a C-section?
- Is there something wrong with me?
- Am I not strong enough or good enough?

These can create feelings of failure, shame, and guilt. Some women feel that there is something wrong with them or their body and feel inadequate.

THE TRUTH

Giving birth is complicated. Many things can go wrong, and it's **NEVER** the woman's fault. We forget that in the past the mortality rate for women and babies during delivery was far higher. Those women didn't have some flaw or do anything wrong; it's just the fact that childbirth has risks. C-sections have lowered that risk considerably, saving lives of both moms and babies.

NO person should ever feel bad about the way they give birth. Every woman who even tries to have a baby is incredible! They are brave, strong, and loving for even making the effort.

TIPS FOR DITCHING THE GUILT

GET CLEAR IN YOUR HEAD

It is important to have a clear perspective about pregnancy. Medical circumstances made it necessary to have a C-section; you didn't do anything wrong.

FORGET ABOUT OTHER PEOPLE

Stop worrying what other people think—how you have your baby is your decision, along with your health-care provider, and no one else's business.

GET SUPPORT

Having a positive and supportive team in place is very important, from your family and friends to your health-care providers, midwife, and doula. Consider a C-section support group, where you can get support from other moms who have had C-sections.

CONCENTRATE ON BONDING

Focus on bonding with your baby when you finally have the opportunity. Skin to skin and bonding with your baby is not about a specific time; it's about being with your baby.

FOCUS ON THE POSITIVE

You and your baby are alive; realize that having the C-section helped you avoid a potentially tragic outcome.

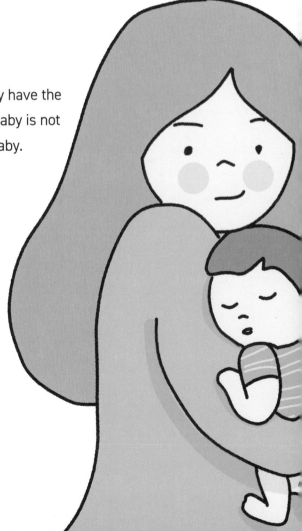

TIME

All things fade with time; know that these feelings will too—so be patient with yourself.

STOP NEGATIVE SELF-TALK

Stop second guessing or beating yourself up. Negative self talk does you no good.

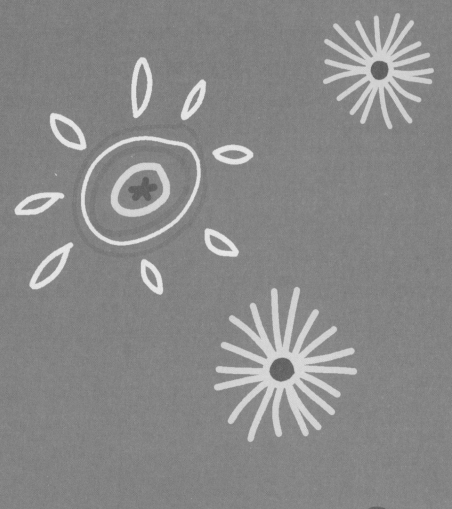

NOTE TO NEW MOMS

Hey, Mom-to-be,

Congratulations—I'm so excited for you!

You may be filled with all kinds of emotions, from joy and happiness to worry and fear. Being pregnant is life changing—literally. You are on one of the most extraordinary journeys of your life.

You may be wondering what kind of mom you're going to be, or if you can even do it. We believe in you and know you can—you will be a great mom.

Will you make mistakes? Of course, everyone does. We all want to do everything right, but it's important to understand that there is no such thing as a perfect parent. We all learn to be the best parent we can be.

Don't be afraid to ask questions or ask for help. Ditch any guilt you might feel—if you are having trouble, ask someone how they dealt with it. You'll be surprised how many moms experience the very same challenges you do but are too afraid to say anything. Your baby and you are too important to let any fear keep you from getting what you need, want, and deserve.

Again, you are amazing, unique, and will be that beautiful light for your child. Sending you all our love and encouragement.

You Got This!
The **SIMPLEST** team

INDEX

<u>Now</u> is the time to prepare for baby's first year!

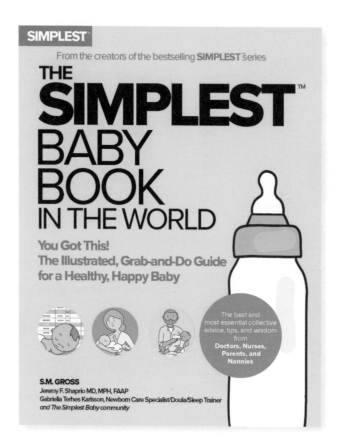

The new must-have parent resource to simplify the first year!

Having a baby can be complex and stressful. *The Simplest Baby Book* makes bringing up baby easier while helping to reduce the stress and creating the confidence to raise a healthy, happy baby, so you can spend more time enjoying what is one of the most magical experiences of your life.

Scan this QR codes for quick access to *The Simplest Baby Book in the World.* Get yours today!

The Illustrated, Grab-and-Do Guide for a Healthy, Happy Baby

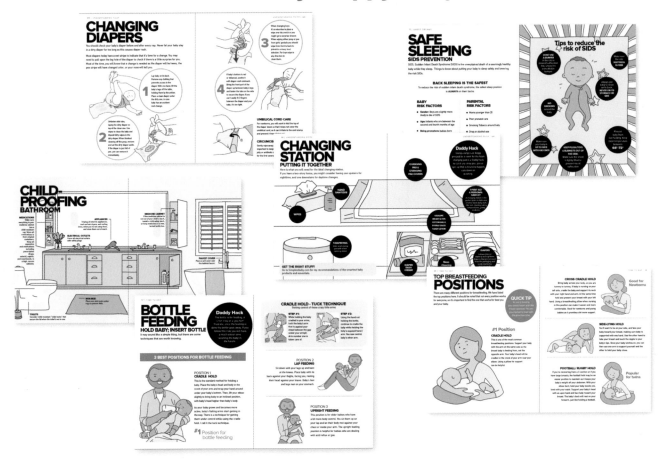

BABY BASICS MADE EASY • INSTANT KNOW-HOW

THE MUST-HAVE LISTS • THE BEST EXPERT ADVICE • BREASTFEEDING 101

GETTING BABY TO SLEEP • INTRODUCING SOLIDS • BABY SAFETY • PARENT TIPS

AND SOOOO MUCH MORE!

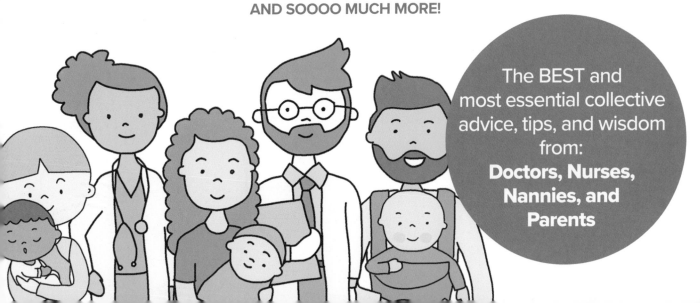

The BEST and most essential collective advice, tips, and wisdom from: Doctors, Nurses, Nannies, and Parents

Limit of Liability/Disclaimer of Warranty: The content of this book is for informational purposes only. The author, publisher and each individual who has made a contribution to the development and production of this book and its contents do not intend this book to be used as medical or other professional advice, and the book is not intended as a substitute for consultation with a licensed practitioner. This book is not intended to replace advice given to you by your and/or your child's physician, and any decisions concerning care are between you and your and/or your child's doctor. Please consult with your or your child's physician or healthcare specialist regarding the suggestions made in this book The publisher, the author and each individual who has made a contribution to the development and production of this book and its contents make no representations or warranties of any kind with respect to this book or its contents, and disclaim all such representations and warranties, express or implied. The examples provided in this book may not apply to the average reader, and are not intended to represent or guarantee that you will achieve the same or similar results. The publisher, the author each individual who has made a contribution to the development and production of this book and its contents assume no responsibility for errors, inaccuracies, omissions, or any other inconsistencies herein, and your use of this book implies your acceptance of this disclaimer.

All the text and artwork in this book are copyright © 2023 Simplest Company LLC. This book or any portion thereof may not be reproduced, stored in a retrieval system, or transmitted, in any form or by any means, electronic, mechanical, photocopying, recording or distributing any part of it in any form without prior written permission from the publisher.

Copyright © 2023 Simplest Company LLC.
All rights reserved.

For more information and product recommendations check out our websites:

simplestbaby.com
simplestpregnancy.com

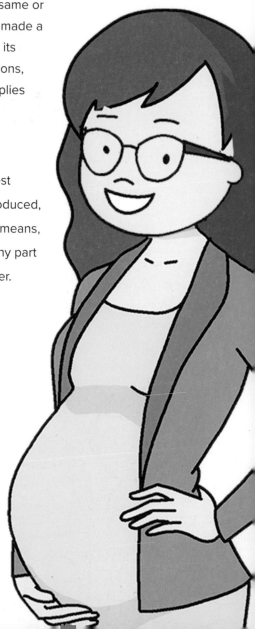